IMAGES
of America

ESSEX COUNTY
OVERBROOK HOSPITAL

IMAGES
of America

ESSEX COUNTY
OVERBROOK HOSPITAL

Kevin R. Kowalick and Kathryn Cataldo
Foreword by Robert L. Williams

ARCADIA
PUBLISHING

Published by Arcadia Publishing
Charleston, South Carolina

Printed in the United States of America

Library of Congress Control Number: 2017937074

For all general information, please contact Arcadia Publishing:
Telephone 843-853-2070
Fax 843-853-0044
E-mail sales@arcadiapublishing.com
For customer service and orders:
Toll-Free 1-888-313-2665

Visit us on the Internet at www.arcadiapublishing.com

*This book is dedicated to the spirit of Overbrook and
the impression that it and its employees made on
mental health care and the local community.*

CONTENTS

FOREWORD

Located below the ridge of the Second Mountain and extending east toward Grove Avenue stood the many buildings of the Essex County Hospital, otherwise known as Overbrook (due to its location west of the Peckman River). The institution was established in Cedar Grove late in the 19th century as a result of overcrowding at the initial complex in Newark. Beginning with the Star Building, with its Victorian-era design and beautiful arched windows, the campus was soon expanded with a series of structures known as the "Hill Buildings."

Although some misinformed thrill seekers have tried to vilify this institution, as the local historian who has studied Overbrook extensively, I can tell you that it was an amazing place that made significant strides in helping those with mental illness, with many caring people on its staff who worked tirelessly to make a positive difference with those in its care. That is not to say that bad things did not happen there, but those that did were the exception to the rule, to be sure.

Overbrook was a city unto itself, complete with its own farm, dairy, train station, rail siding with storehouses, and power plant. Besides the many wards in the different buildings, there were buildings that housed nurses, an auditorium, fire stations, and the superintendent's mansion, to name of few others.

Many of these buildings, with their beautiful period architecture, stood proudly for over a century. However, as the wheels of time continued to turn, county politicians decided to close the place after building a modern facility nearby. The ensuing years found these buildings as abandoned relics crying out for preservation and re-use, but those cries fell on deaf ears.

The county sold the complex after stripping away some of its architectural beauty, and one by one, the buildings, with their tunnels, were removed with yet again another missed opportunity for historic preservation and saving the best of our cultural heritage.

In his book, Kevin Kowalick delves into the history of Overbrook and explains its storied past. He, like so many others, explored the abandoned complex and was captivated by its history, architecture, and the many relics left behind. As you read through the pages of this book, I am certain you will encounter Kevin's passion for this special place and his desire that the stories of Overbrook, and the people associated with it, not be forgotten.

—Robert L. Williams
Historian

ACKNOWLEDGMENTS

The authors would like to give special thanks to Robert L. Williams, Carl Franzetti, Mark Miller, Frank J. DelGaudio, Kathy Kauhl, and George Hawley. Without your contributions and accommodations, creating this book would have been impossible.

We would also like to thank Brian Holbig for his plethora of knowledge regarding historical sites in New Jersey, as well as our many friends, including Julia Rivera, Karlee King, Dylan Volb, Patrick McClernan, Dan Karcher, Pat Hayes, Justin Gurbisz, Frank Koch, Ryan Maron, Brett Begovich, Heidi Steffan, Michael Helbing, Michael Clark, Lisa Blohm, Matt Smith, Tina Hammersmark, Christina Mathews, Rusty Tagliareni, and Matthew Todd. Matt was a great friend to all and unexpectedly passed away shortly before this book came to be. We have shared many years of fun memories seeking out the next big adventure. His infectious laugh and amazing sense of humor will be greatly missed.

Unless otherwise noted, all images appear courtesy of Essex County, New Jersey.

To me, Kevin Kowalick, Overbrook has always been much more than a complex of rotting buildings sitting in the beautiful suburbs of Cedar Grove, New Jersey. When I first visited the complex almost six years ago now, I was instantly drawn in. Overbrook was a place that piqued my curiosity over the edge of looking at it through a computer screen. I could not explain the connection that drew me to Overbrook so strongly. I became fascinated with its lore and history. I found myself spending countless hours researching and photographing the historic site. I hope that with the completion of this book, Kathryn and I will preserve the spirit of Overbrook forever.

INTRODUCTION

The Essex County Overbrook Hospital opened its doors in December 1898. The hospital opened as a single building, the Star Building, and a small powerhouse located behind it. In the years to come, the hospital would expand to what was known as the largest county hospital in the state of New Jersey. Operating with over 50 buildings, Overbrook served as a town in itself and had every necessary amenity to be self-sustaining. Many firsts in both medical history and New Jersey history came from Overbrook and its operations. The hospital became a prominent landmark not only in Verona and Cedar Grove but also in Essex County as a whole. Although the treatment of mental illness in a typical asylum setting was a controversial topic, Overbrook was a prestigious institution that cared for its patients. The iconic brick buildings that were constructed in the early 1900s stood proud for over 100 years as a reminder of history. The hospital slowly started closing wards down as the treatment of psychiatric illness turned toward medications. In 2007, Overbrook officially closed, and patients were moved to the new Essex County Hospital Center on Grove Avenue. The new hospital is much smaller in size, as the need for a 50-building, long-term-stay psychiatric hospital is no more. Overbrook sat vacant from that point on, allowing only the curious to step inside. The employee buildings on the west side of Fairview Avenue were all demolished by 2011. By this time, only a few buildings on the main hospital side of Fairview Avenue had been demolished. The main campus sat in a state of decay and neglect for years to come. In 2015, a deal was made between Essex County and K. Hovnanian to sell the hospital grounds for development of condominium units. From late 2015 onward, history began to slowly disappear in the quiet suburbs of Cedar Grove, New Jersey. Overbrook was to be completely demolished, with no form of preservation or remembrance of over 100 years of history. In this book, we will preserve what Overbrook was and what it did for the community and mental health care. We will take readers from Overbrook's inception to its final days. In between, readers will be familiarized with Overbrook's many buildings, look into how the hospital functioned as a city in itself, meet the staff and patients of the hospital, and learn about the treatments and conditions to which both patients and staff were exposed. The book ends with Overbrook's popular phase of abandonment and its depressing destruction.

One

LAYOUT AND PURPOSE

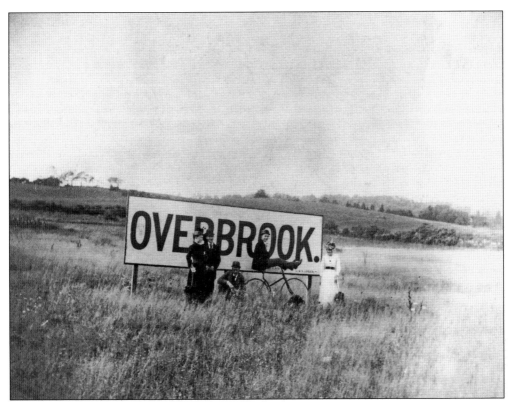

Overbrook began its life as an auxiliary hospital for the Essex County Insane Asylum in Newark, New Jersey. The land was purchased in Verona Township in 1896 with the intention to remedy overcrowding at the main institution. This photograph was taken where the Overbrook property met Grove Avenue. The Grosch family of the American Bronze Powder Mill on Grove Avenue, a prominent family in Verona, is pictured posing with the Overbrook property sign. (Courtesy of Robert L. Williams.)

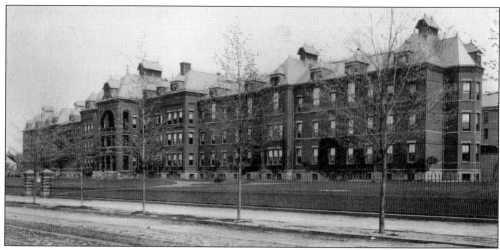

The Essex County Asylum for the Insane was founded in 1872. The asylum was initially located on Camden Street in Newark, New Jersey. The first patients were eight transfers from the nearby Essex County Jail. By 1884, the hospital had moved to a more suitable location on South Orange Avenue in Newark. This was one of the first county-owned hospitals dedicated to mental health in the state. The hospital featured several dormitories that extended out from the main center structure. The institution featured 17 wards, nine being single rooms. Wards 1 and 2 housed double rooms, and the rest of the wards were large dormitories. In the mid-1890s, the number of individuals needing mental health care in Essex County was on the rise. The hospital soon began to see overcrowding and outbreaks of community illnesses such as smallpox and dysentery. (Both, courtesy of the Newark Public Library.)

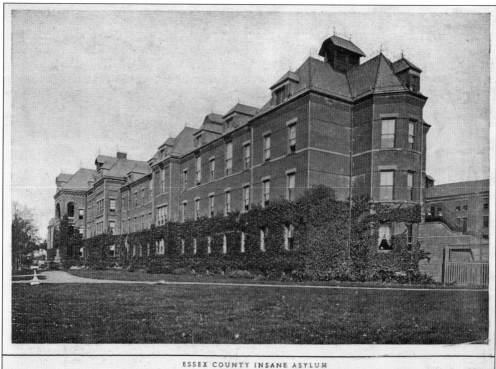

ESSEX COUNTY INSANE ASYLUM
South Orange Avenue.

10

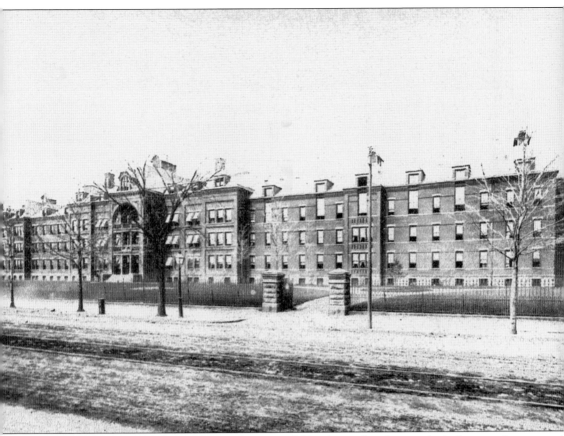

By 1895, the hospital housed 635 patients. There were 257 males, with only enough single rooms for 110. There were 378 females, with only enough single rooms to house 169. This became a serious concern due to the mental condition of the patients. For safety alone, it was recommended that each patient have a single room. The state hospital at Morris Plains, New Jersey, Greystone State Hospital, was also suffering with overcrowding, so no relief could be found in transferring patients there. It was determined that an additional wing to the current hospital would cost $80,000 and provide relief for at most two years. With a prediction of at least 130 patients coming through 1896, a solution needed to be found. It was at this time that the idea of expansion was conceived. (Courtesy of the Newark Public Library.)

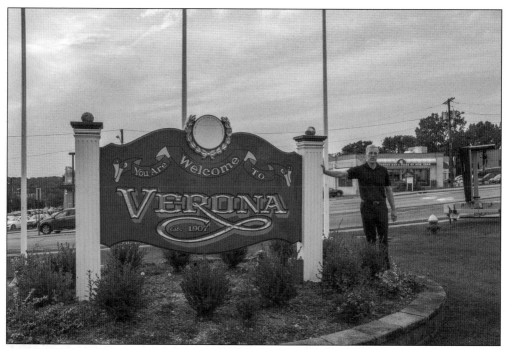

In 1896, the decision was made to purchase a 325-acre plot in Verona Township to erect a new branch hospital. At this time, it was thought that having outdoor therapy services would greatly improve mental health. This was a treatment that could not be preformed at the South Orange Avenue hospital. The location of the branch hospital offered open spaces to accommodate outdoor therapeutic treatments. Robert L. Williams is pictured in front of the Verona town sign. (Photograph by Kevin Kowalick.)

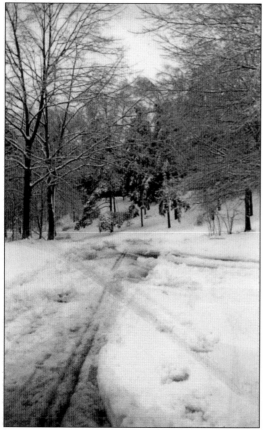

The land on which Overbrook was intended to be built was initially known as Verona Township. What is now known as Cedar Grove Township was once part of Verona Township. Cedar Grove Township was founded in 1908. The first building at Overbrook, the Star Building, became the largest structure in Cedar Grove.

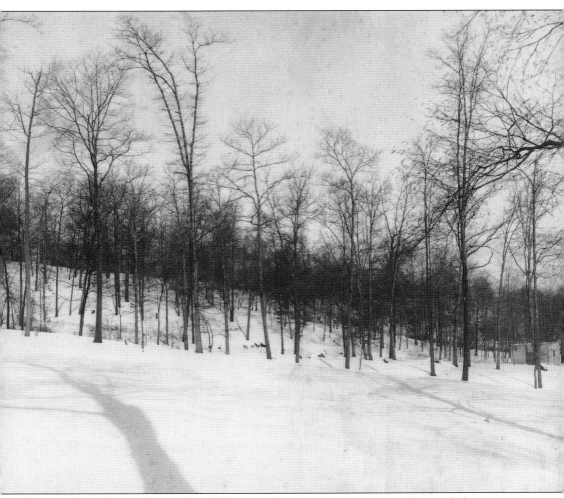

The grounds at the new hospital would feature a large open area between the wooded sections. This area would soon be determined as the recreational field for patient and staff actives. It would feature a bandstand for concerts, a baseball field, and a volleyball net. The campus was built into the side of a mountain, thus offering a unique layout to the hospital. The location proved to be exactly what hospital officials and the board of chosen freeholders wanted. Construction did not delay, and soon, the parcel of land was being developed.

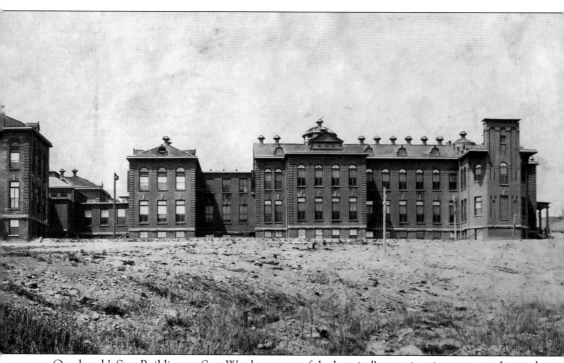

Overbrook's Star Building, or Star Ward, was one of the hospital's most iconic structures. It was the first building constructed in the period of 1896–1897. The Star Building housed wards 1 through 9 and both male and female patients. It was the largest building to ever be constructed on the Overbrook campus. In the beginning years, Overbrook operated as solely the Star Building and the small powerhouse to the east on the other side of the train tracks. On December 18, 1898, the Star Building was occupied, and Overbrook saw its first patients, 102 males and 142 females transferred from the South Orange Avenue facility. The patients were let off at the Overbrook train stop on the Caldwell branch of the Erie Railroad. The brass band of the Newark City Home, under the supervision of Caleb M. Harrison, played somber melodies as the patients embarked up the hill to the Star Building. In 1910, the South Orange Avenue facility closed, and the rest of the patients were transferred to Overbrook in four days—200 patients per day. (Courtesy of Robert L. Williams.)

The next group of buildings constructed were known as the Hill Buildings. The structures were on top of a hill that overlooked the Star Building, the athletic field, and the valley between Second and First Mountain. These buildings were the iconic red and whitish yellow brick cottages that became associated with Overbrook. Construction began in 1905, when it was decided that more space was needed. By 1909, most of the Hill Buildings were completed.

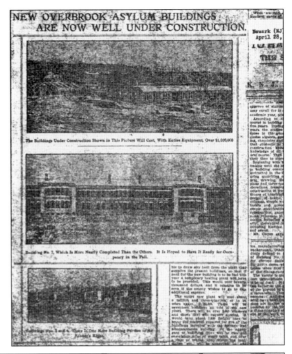

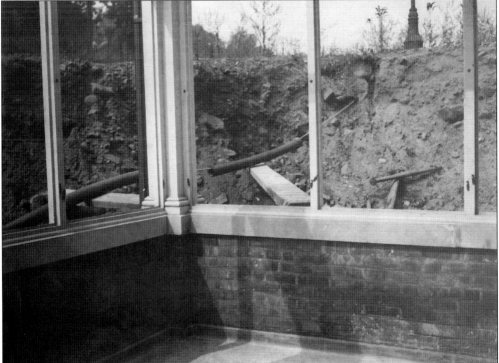

The photograph above shows the challenges faced during the construction of the hospital. The mountainside needed to be dug out in order for the buildings to have a flat foundation. The campus was divided into three different levels, each having to be dug out of the eastern slope of Second Mountain. (Courtesy of the Newark Public Library.)

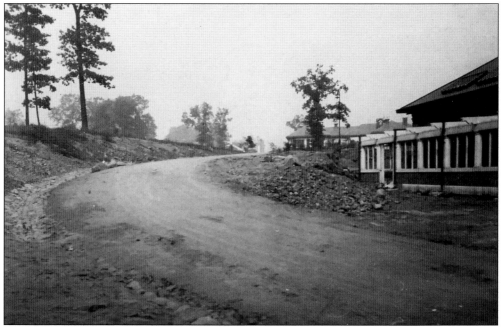

Overbrook sat on the eastern slope of Second Mountain above the Peckman River. The Peckman River starts in West Orange, New Jersey, and runs north to the Passaic River. This is where the name "Overbrook" originated—the campus sat over the brook, the Peckman River. The river later became a spot for the hospital's livestock to drink fresh water from during the agricultural phase of the hospital.

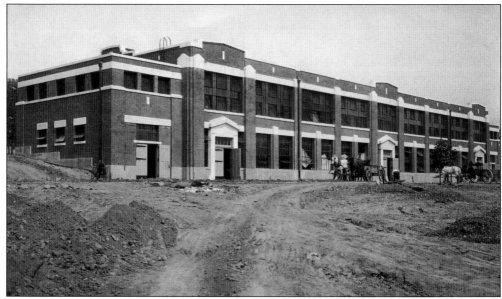

In the 1895 annual report book, it was discussed that there was a need for more occupational and recreational therapies used as forms of treatment. Open space and room for more recreational therapies was a main factor in purchasing the land in Verona Township. By 1910, the Occupational Therapy Building was completed, and it served as a place for patients to participate in different forms of hands-on activities. (Courtesy of the Newark Public Library.)

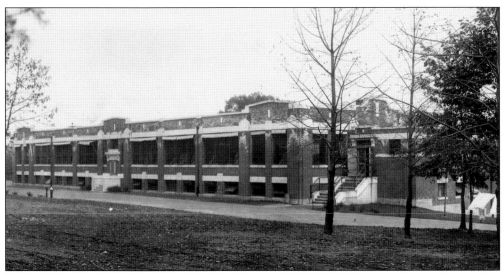

This building became a key part of Overbrook's functionality and treatment of patients. In 1960, Clive Krygar, director of the occupational therapy unit, represented the hospital at the Annual Conference of the American Occupational Therapy Association. The occupational therapy department held annual fairs and was hosted at local Essex County events. The department also offered programs for students in local colleges and universities to perform internships at the hospital.

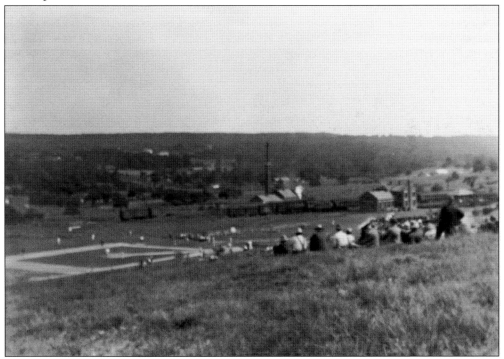

A different angle of the open space shows the area after being developed. The baseball field can be seen, with patients and staff sitting atop the hill watching the game. In the background, the hospital's original powerhouse can be seen with a train passing by the front of it. The building in front of the train was the hospital's pathology building.

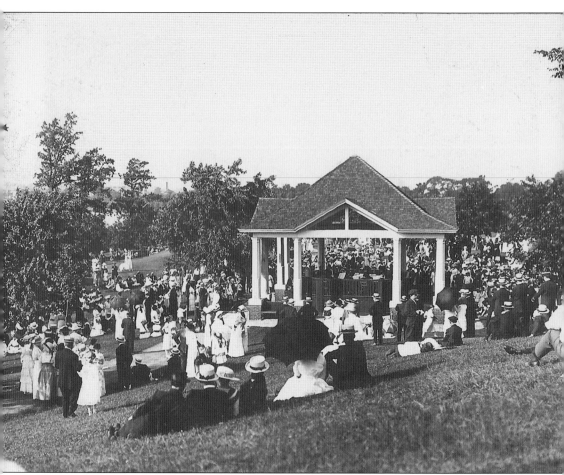

This view shows the pavilion, or bandstand, in the early 20th century. This is an area that patients would frequently visit during months in which they were able to be outdoors. Around 150 patients were allowed on the grounds unattended. Each patient had to carry a card citing his or her limits and time to report back inside. Male patients were allowed to stay out until 9:00 p.m. If hospital patients did not check back in by their given time, hospital staff would be able to track who was missing due to the card they carried along with daily ward checks. Many patients did run off but were caught by local police departments and brought back to the hospital center.

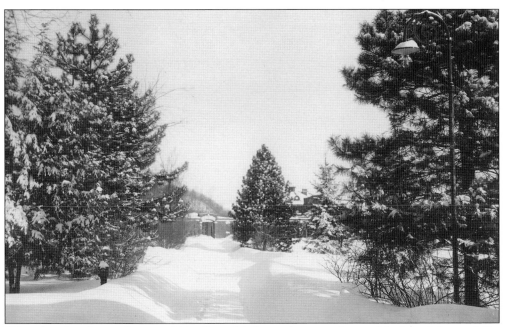

When Overbrook initially opened, Dr. Henry McCormick was in charge of the branch hospital. Dr. Daniel Dill was superintendent at the South Orange Avenue facility and later became superintendent at Overbrook in 1901. Both doctors were advocates for open space and tranquil environments at Overbrook, as seen in the photograph above. (Courtesy of Robert L. Williams.)

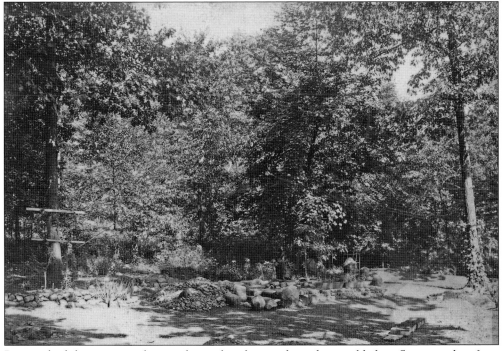

Patients had their own outdoor garden and craft area where they could plant flowers and preform other gardening activities. This was thought to be a form of therapy, and Overbrook provided plenty of open space for the psychologists to administer this type of occupational treatment.

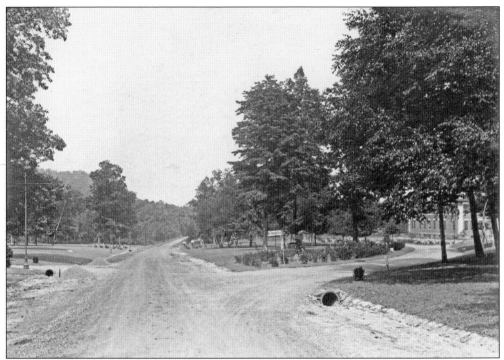

Fairview Avenue is the main road that connects Verona to Cedar Grove today. This is the road that Overbrook was built on. The Administration Building sat on the road, with the ward buildings set back from it. The photograph above features Fairview Avenue in 1914 with Ward Building 5 seen in the distance to the right.

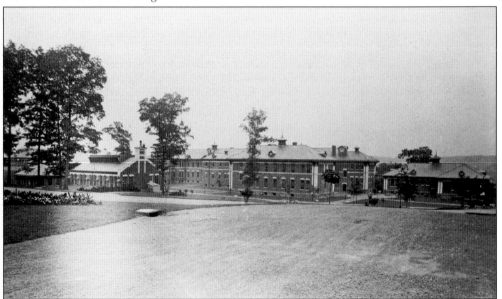

This photograph was taken from the west side of Fairview Avenue. Fairview Avenue cut Overbrook's campus in half. The terms "east side of Fairview" and "west side of Fairview" were commonly used in reference to the hospital in the annual reports. The view above is looking onto the east side of campus from the west side of campus. Hill Building 1 and the main kitchen can be seen.

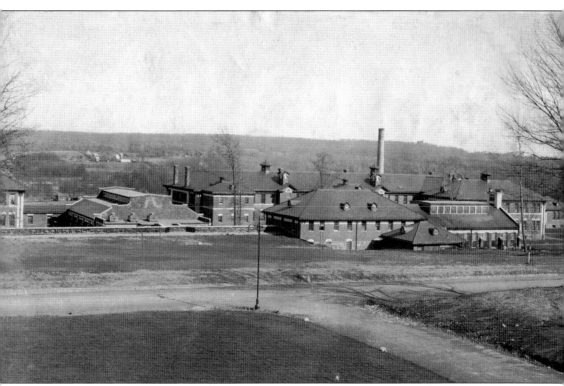

This photograph is a great example of how the campus was set up. Ward Building 1 is the largest building in the background. The building closest to Fairview Avenue is the kitchen; to the left of the kitchen is Dining Hall 9. Each ward building has a small, single-story hallway that connects to the next building. One hallway can be seen to the left of the dining hall connecting to Ward Building 2. Their main purpose was so that staff and patients could move from building to building without having to go outside or into the basement tunnel system. The system of aboveground walkways connected all the main Hill Buildings on campus. During the hospital's period of modernization in later years, elevated breezeways were introduced to connect Administration to Hill Building 3 and Hill Building 3 to the Reception Building. (Courtesy of Robert L. Williams.)

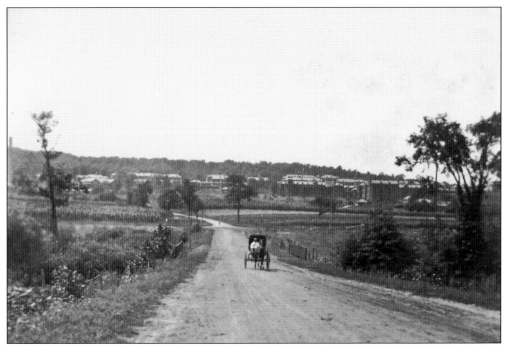

Bradford Avenue was, and still is, another main roadway in Cedar Grove. This road cut across First Mountain and connected Upper Montclair to Cedar Grove. It had one of the best views of the hospital center. Both of these photographs were taken from Bradford Avenue looking at the Overbrook campus around 1914. The Overbrook property extended across Bradford Avenue; this is where the main agricultural activity of the hospital center took place. Crops were planted along both sides of the road, which can be seen in both photographs, and were harvested as food for patients at the hospital. (Both, courtesy of Robert L. Williams.)

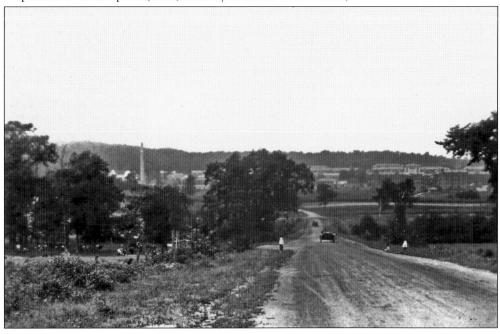

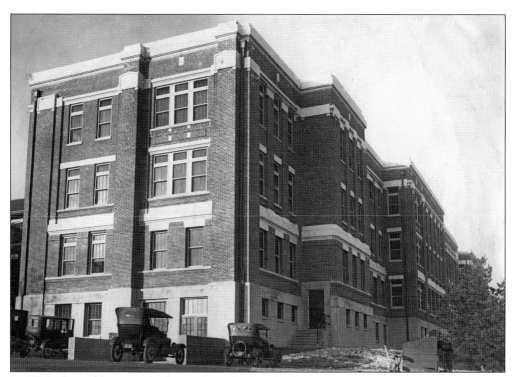

In 1925, a key addition to the hospital was built—the Reception Building, or Building 11. The Reception Building played a key role in the hospital's functions. This is where everyone admitted to the hospital was brought to be checked in. It served as the main medical building, housing the hospital's only surgical suites. An addition costing $418,827 was made to the Reception Building in 1960 to attempt to alleviate overcrowding by adding 42 new beds. In later days, the building was used to house the more dangerous patients on campus. This building featured its own dining area, exam rooms, and dorm rooms so the more dangerous patients were not mixed in with the rest. The Reception Building was home to the medical testing laboratories and the morgue when the main pathology building was shut down. (Above, courtesy of the Newark Public Library.)

Break Ground At Overbrook

—— NEWS

Reception Building at Hospital to Cost $418,827 OCT 4

Ground was broken yesterday for a $418,827 addition to the reception building at the Essex County Hospital at Cedar Grove (Overbrook).

Freeholder James L. McKenna, chairman of the board of free-holders' hospitals' committee, presided at the ceremony. He said the new addition would alleviate crowding at the institution, whose population, according to Dr. Henry A. Davidson, superintendent and medical director, reached a record 3,860 during September.

The federal government is contributing $118,000 toward the total cost. The three-story addition will provide 42 new beds, interview rooms for both doctors and social workers, and a new diet kitchen.

The addition is the second stage of the 1960 building program. A one million dollar wing is being added to the administration building.

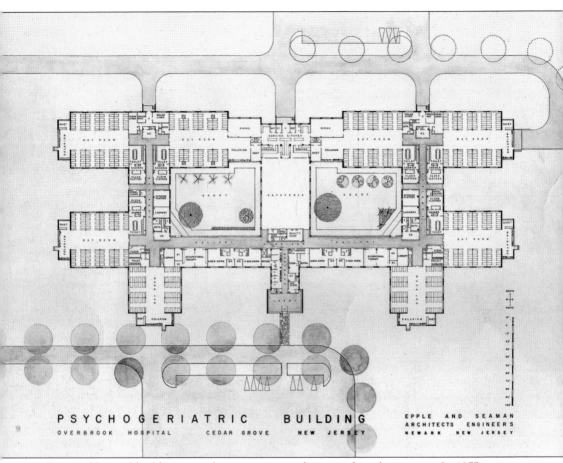

PSYCHOGERIATRIC BUILDING

OVERBROOK HOSPITAL   CEDAR GROVE   NEW JERSEY

EPPLE AND SEAMAN
ARCHITECTS ENGINEERS
NEWARK   NEW JERSEY

Soon, additional buildings were being constructed to complete the campus. In 1957, a geriatrics building was constructed. At this time, the hospital had predominantly geriatric patients; 24 percent of patients over the age of 80 were considered senile. It was imperative to have a special program for geriatrics. The Wright Pavilion (Psychogeriatric Building) was built and dedicated to this purpose. Above are the blueprints. Epple and Seaman were the architects. This company was based out of Newark and was prominent in architecture during this time. The building was constructed on Grove Avenue, the road running parallel to Fairview Avenue at the south end of campus. The building still exists as Alaris Health at Cedar Grove, a nursing care facility.

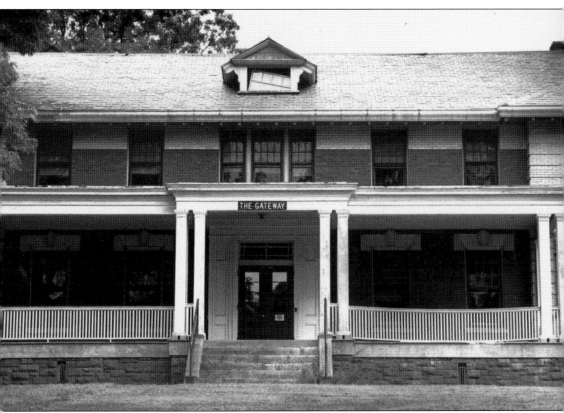

As the hospital grew, it offered more services in different buildings on campus. Gateway was opened in 1965 as a halfway house between the institution and the community. The building was converted from former staff housing. The Gateway Building featured 21 rooms, all of them single private rooms. The patients were given keys to their own rooms, which gave them physical evidence of their improvement from being in Overbrook's main wards. Fifteen women were chosen as the first patients to occupy the Gateway Building. They ranged in age from 20 to 50 years old and were patients at Overbrook anywhere from six months to five years. The plan for the institution was to add patients every two weeks until all 21 beds in Gateway were filled. (Courtesy of the Newark Public Library.)

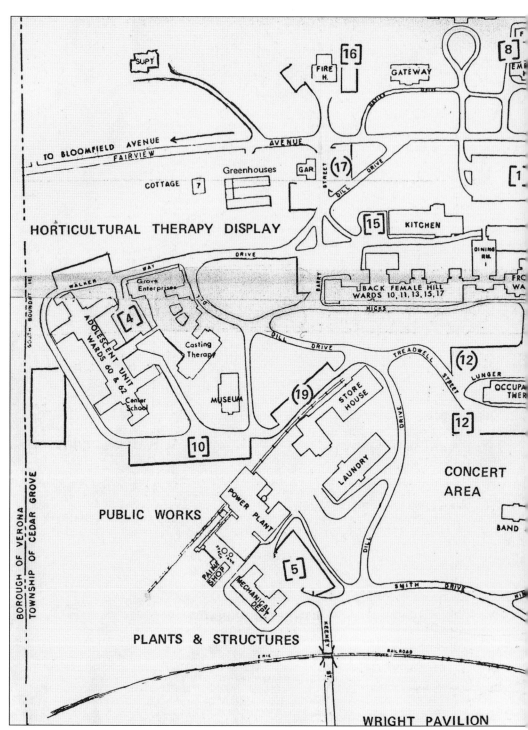

This is a map of the hospital center dating to the mid-1950s. This is the most complete map of Overbrook before certain buildings were demolished and demonstrates how Fairview Avenue runs across the property, splitting the campus in two. Above Fairview Avenue is where all the nurses' and doctors' homes, auditorium, firehouse, and various administrative buildings were located. Below

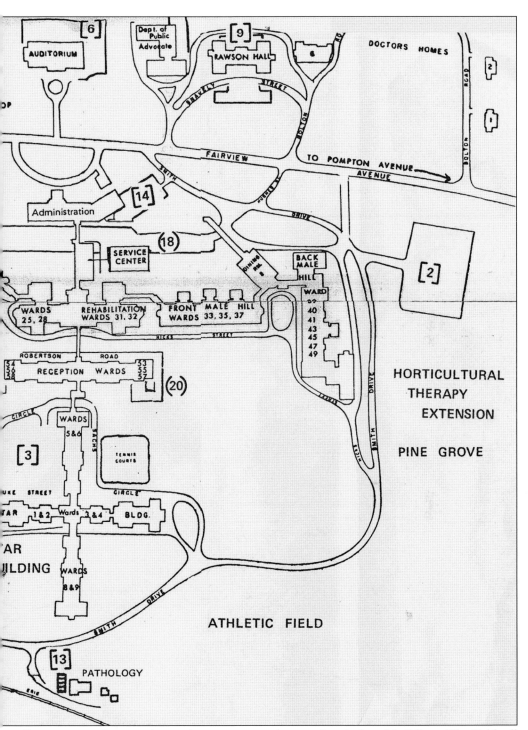

Fairview were the main hospital center, power plant, and agricultural buildings. The Caldwell Branch of the Erie Railroad can be seen running below the main hospital complex. A station for the Overbrook Hospital was located next to the pathology building. Below the railroad tracks was where the Wright Pavilion and farmhouse stood.

27

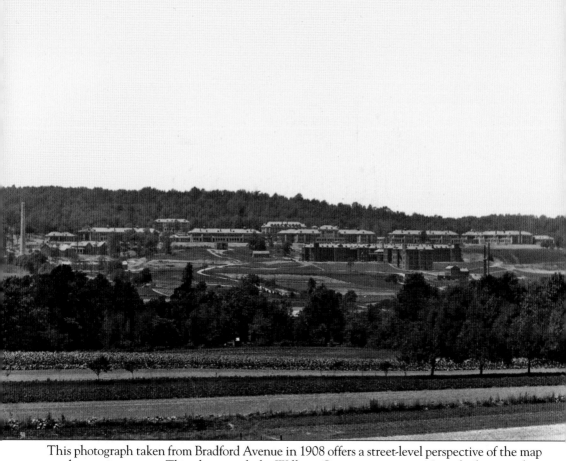

This photograph taken from Bradford Avenue in 1908 offers a street-level perspective of the map on the previous pages. This photograph, by William Cone, a prominent Newark photographer, also illustrates how the campus sat on the mountain face of Second Mountain. The building farthest to the back and left was the female employees' home across Fairview Avenue. To the right of that, the back of Administration can be seen. Behind Administration are, from left to right, Hill Ward Buildings 1 through 5. Below the Hill Wards sits the Star Ward, the largest building on campus. To the left of the Star Ward by the woods are the powerhouse, mechanics shop, and storehouse. The building directly to the east of the Star Ward is the pathology building. Finally, the smokestack that can be seen coming from the woods is the original powerhouse for the facility. Note that the Reception Building is missing between Hill Ward Three and the Star Building, as the photograph was taken before 1925. (Courtesy of the Newark Public Library.)

Two

BUILDINGS AND STRUCTURES

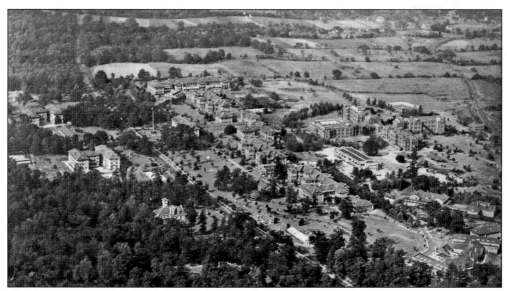

The Essex County Overbrook Hospital was the largest county-run hospital center in the state of New Jersey. The property spanned 640 acres, with 53 buildings on the hospital grounds at one time. The hospital became one of the largest employers in Essex County. In the early 1900s, nearly 820 staff members were working at the hospital center in some way. By 1909, Overbrook was cited as the most modern mental facility in the country. The hospital soon became a significant part of history, not only because of its impact on mental health care but also for its impact on the local economy. (Courtesy of the Newark Public Library.)

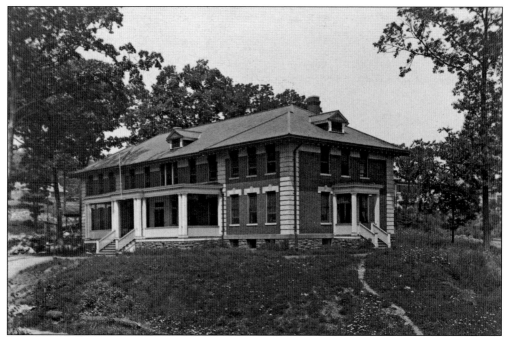

Pictured is one of the staff cottages at Overbrook. These buildings had similar architecture to the ward buildings. Most of the employee housing was constructed on the west side of Fairview Avenue. This particular building was the only staff housing on the east side of Fairview Avenue with the main hospital buildings. Hill Building 1 can be seen behind and to the right. The original firehouse can be seen in the back to the left.

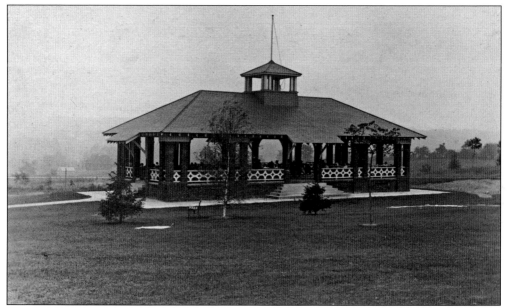

The bandstand was located in the field in front of the Star Building. This structure was used as a space for patients to sit outside and enjoy the weather. Scheduled music events were also featured here. The hospital had its own music department, which regularly held concerts here, weather permitting.

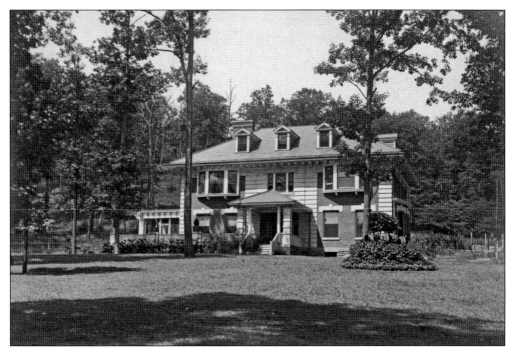

The superintendent's home was among the group of buildings on the west side of Fairview Avenue. Matching the red and whitish yellow brick architecture of the Hill Wards, this home was built in the early 1900s for the superintendent of the hospital. The building's opulent interior featured paneled oak woodwork, a grand oak staircase, and stained and leaded glass windows.

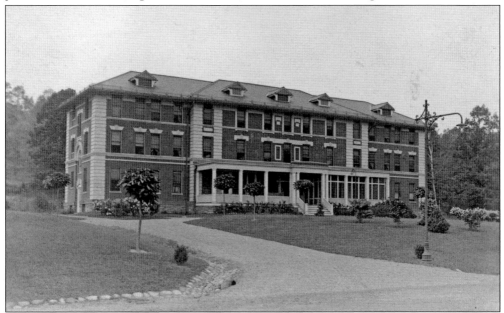

The female employees' home on the west side of Fairview Avenue was one of the largest faculty housing buildings at Overbrook. This three-story, cottage-style dormitory consisted of small apartment-like living spaces, with shared bathrooms, kitchens, and living rooms. An underground tunnel ran from this building under Fairview Avenue to the main campus.

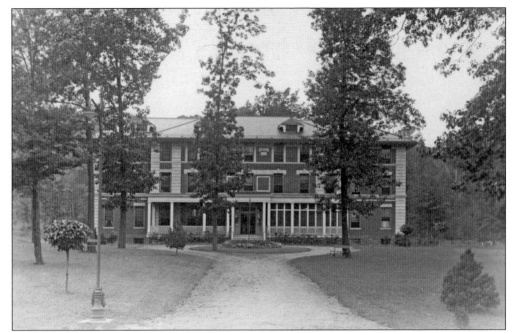

The student nurses' home sat slightly behind and to the left of the female employees' home. This building was designated for the students of the Essex County Hospital Center's Training School for Nurses. The training school was established in 1886 and soon became a destination for student nurses to train from across the nation.

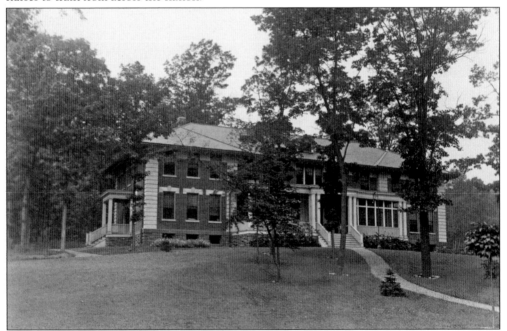

Employee cottages were not the only use for the buildings on the west side of Fairview Avenue. Some buildings were used by different agencies in the hospital. Most of the structures that started out as employee cottages were eventually converted for other uses. For example, the department of public advocacy for the hospital was located here.

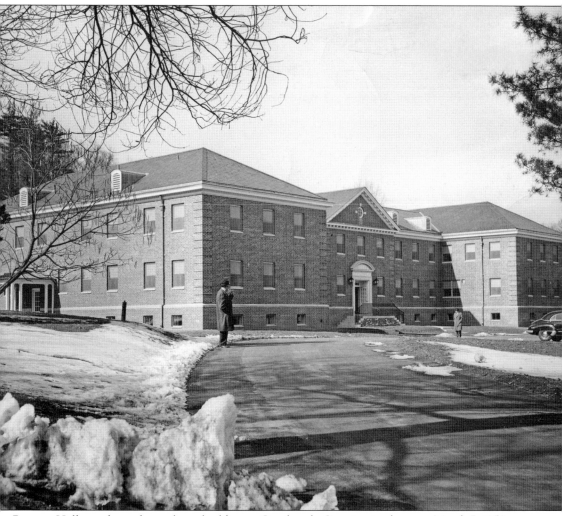

Rawson Hall was the male employee building at Overbrook. Opening its doors on March 7, 1950, the building was part of an ongoing plan to bring more employee housing on campus. The cost of the two-story structure was $485,000. This particular building was intended to attract "high class employees" to the hospital center. Rawson Hall consisted of 11 two-room living apartments on its first floor. This accommodated space for four doctors, a supervisor, and the choice of either six married couples or 12 male employees. Kitchens, bathrooms, and a lounge area were provided on this floor as well. The second floor of the building housed 38 individual rooms. The building came fully furnished with maple furniture in individual rooms and red and green metal tube chairs in the lounge rooms. (Courtesy of the Newark Public Library.)

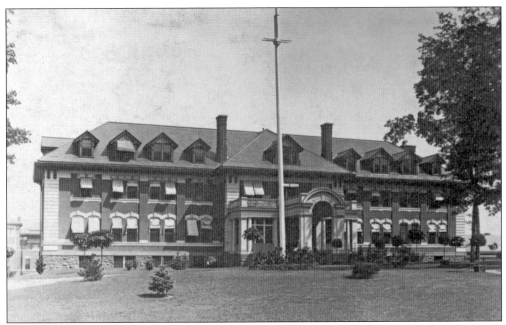

The Administration Building at Overbrook was one of the most iconic buildings on campus. This 1914 view shows the original arched entry structure, which became three arched structures in 1960. This building housed all the staff that kept the hospital functioning. Everything from accounting to security operated here.

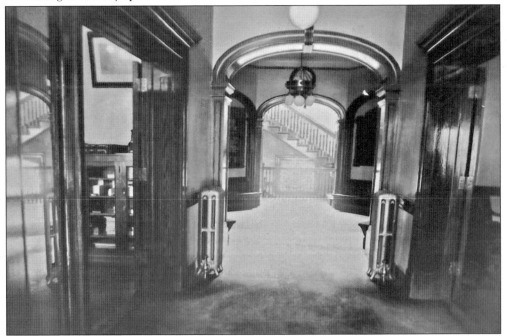

This 1914 photograph gives an interior look at Administration, or Building 6. The building contained the most elegant interior design on campus. The main staircase can be seen at the end of the hallway. Before the staircase, a bronze plaque can be seen to the right that listed important figures in Overbrook's history up to the time period when the Hill Buildings were built.

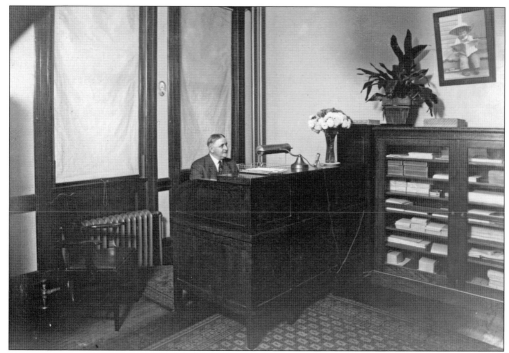

This photograph shows a typical office room inside the Administration Building. The clerk's department was one of the most vital organizations housed in the building. In 1912, this department installed a system of index cards in alphabetical order that covered patients' admissions, discharges, and deaths. A record of a patient's personal belongings was kept on a separate notecard and attached to the main card.

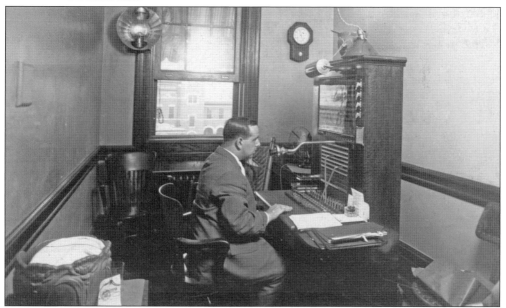

The main operator was housed inside the Administration Building. All the calls into the hospital center came through here. If a family member were calling in to speak with a patient, it would first come to this office, and the operator would transfer the call to the appropriate party.

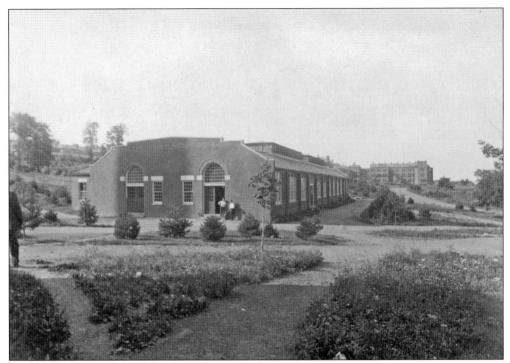

Seen here is a 1914 view of the side of the laundry building. The laundry building was in close proximity to the powerhouse. The hospital had separate buildings such as a soap factory and mattress shop for more specific items.

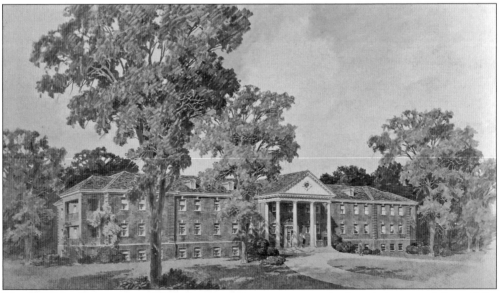

The PEER building was used for administrative purposes at the hospital center. Most of the department was dedicated to filing information for the hospital. This included records of hospital expenditures and other financial reports. Once filed in order by date, staff members took the files to the records room to be properly stored. (Courtesy of the Newark Public Library.)

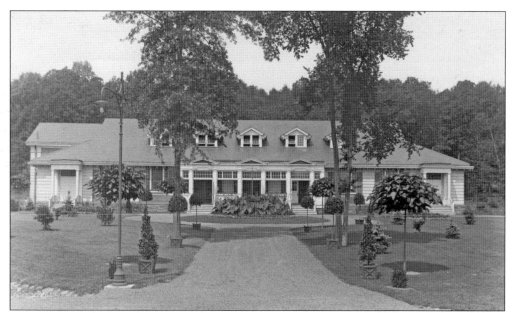

The auditorium was a single-story building on the west side of Fairview Avenue alongside the employee homes. It was commonly referred to as Assembly Hall in early years and the Guy Payne Auditorium in later years. This open structure was designated for staff and patient events and entertainment. Before the chapel was constructed in the service building, Building 7, in 1951, this was where religious services were held. Patients put on plays year-round as well as musical performances in winter months and in inclement weather. Dances and movies were held weekly for a nine-month period. The building was one of the only ones at Overbrook that was open to the public for regular events held by the hospital. The building was also used by other groups and enterprises in Cedar Grove that had no affiliation with the hospital center. The building was demolished in 1970s.

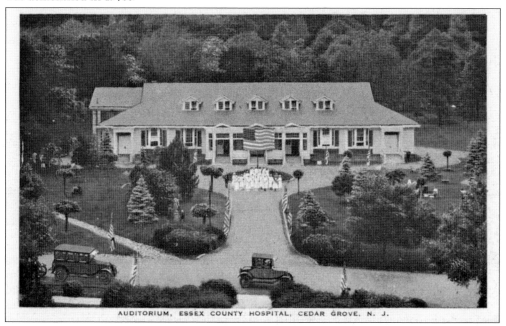

AUDITORIUM, ESSEX COUNTY HOSPITAL, CEDAR GROVE, N. J.

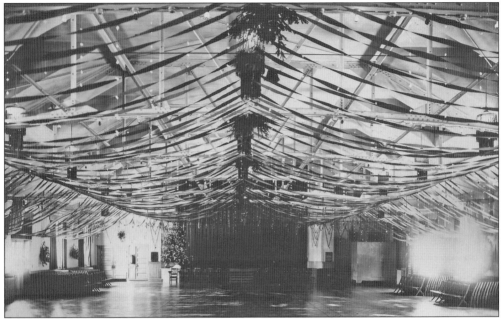

The interior of the auditorium was decorated for each event. It was also decorated for seasonal holiday celebrations. It was a one-level auditorium set up with folding chairs when seating was available for events. In this photograph, the building is decorated for Christmas.

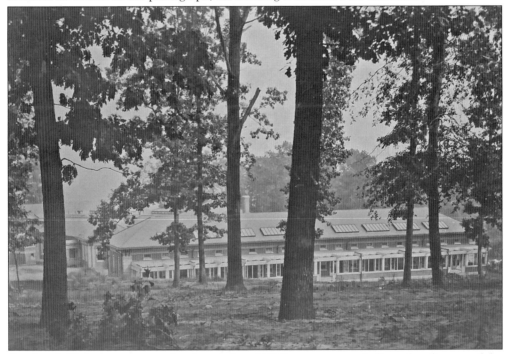

Overbrook felt it was necessary for there to be a building on campus dedicated to diseases of the chest, especially tuberculosis. This building was opened on August 23, 1916. In 1953, after the operation of the Essex Mountain Sanatorium, this building was known as the Freeman Pavilion. The Freeman Pavilion held both adolescent wards and county facilities such as Grove Enterprises.

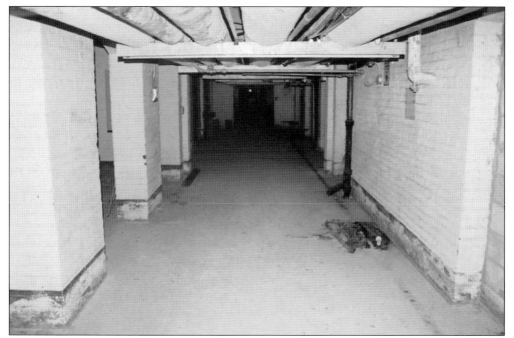

Another grouping of smaller buildings was to the south of the main hospital campus. These were the service and maintenance buildings. These key buildings kept the hospital operating at maximum efficiency. Included in this group were the powerhouse and laundry buildings. A system of underground tunnels connected these to the main campus so workers could easily service any issues, as seen above in the basement of one of the wards. (Courtesy of Robert L. Williams.)

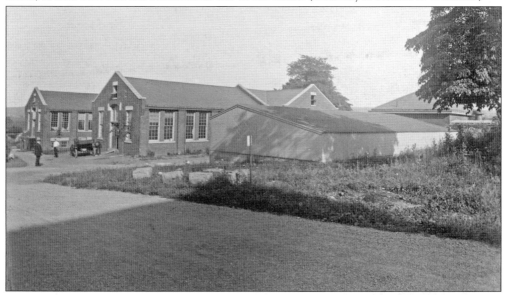

A 1914 view shows the mechanics shop, located next to the powerhouse building. This building is where much of the maintenance work for the hospital was done. Hospital employees in this building were responsible for the general upkeep of the hospital buildings. The locksmith for the grounds was also in this building. Each individual ward had a specific key, although a master key had the ability to unlock any door in the entire hospital.

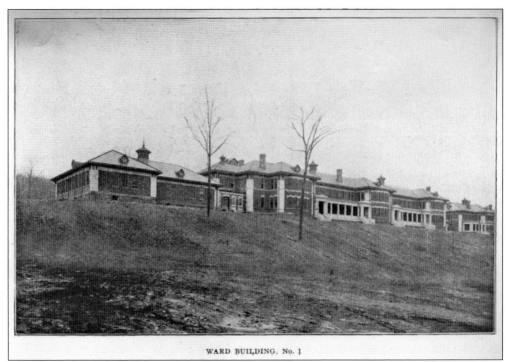

WARD BUILDING, No. 1

Hill Building 1 was the Back Female Ward Building, housing Wards 10 through 17. This building had two additional structures attached to it. One was designated for Ward 10, which can be seen on the left side of the building. The other, in the back of the building, was for Ward 11. Both wards were shut down before the rest of the wards in this building. (Courtesy of Robert L. Williams.)

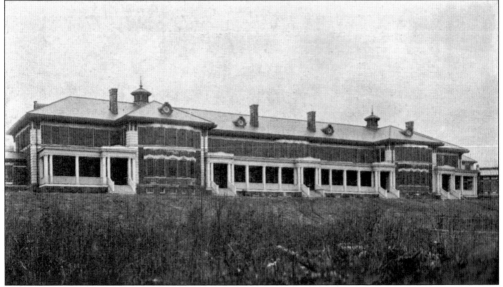

Hill Building 2 was designated as the Front Female Ward Building; it consisted of Wards 19 through 23. All of the Hill Buildings were constructed between 1905 and 1909. This particular building, along with Hill Building 1, was designated for female patients only with no age specifications. (Courtesy of Robert L. Williams.)

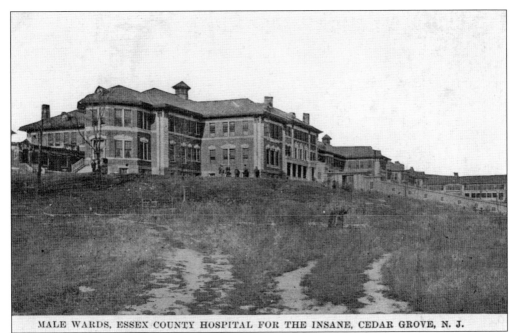

MALE WARDS, ESSEX COUNTY HOSPITAL FOR THE INSANE, CEDAR GROVE, N. J.

Hill Building 3 was unique and served as the center of the campus. It was initially set up as male wards and later designated as the Rehabilitation Wards, housing Wards 25, 28, 31, and 32. This building featured workout equipment, hydrotherapy, and the hospital's main records rooms. There were three records rooms in the basement. This building was also mixed with wards and employee offices. A small hallway connected this to the Star Building before the Reception Wards were built in 1925. (Courtesy of Robert L. Williams.)

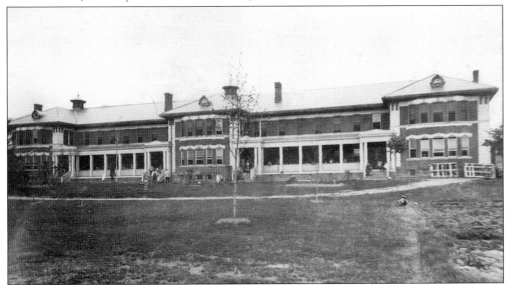

Hill Buildings 4 and 5 were designated as the male wards. Hill Building 4 was the Front Male Wards, and No. 5 was the Back Male Wards. Pictured here is Hill Building 5, the only building to not sit on a northward facing line. The other structure jetting off from the main ward was later known as the MICA Ward. This ward specifically treated the mentally ill and chemically addicted patients. (Courtesy of Robert L. Williams.)

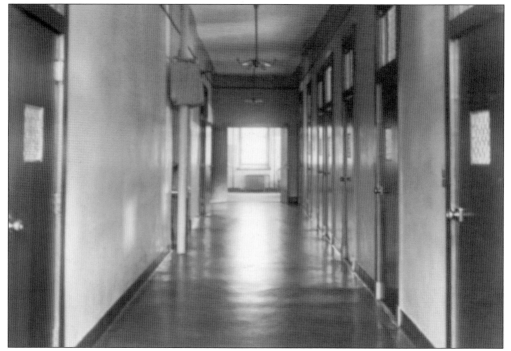

This is an example of the interior of one of the hill wards. This typical ward had multiple single-patient rooms and one seclusion room. This particular building is Hill Building 2. Hill Buildings 1, 2, 4, and 5 were very similar. More patient rooms were located on the second floor than the first. Each patient room had a bed, nightstand, and wardrobe. Each room also had a window so that patients were able to see outside.

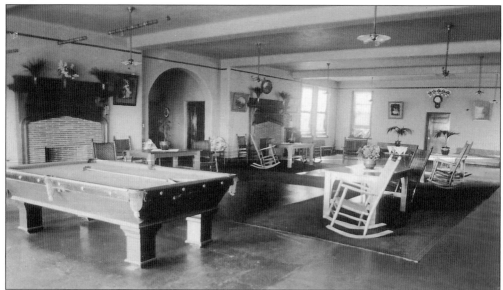

The dayrooms at Overbrook were meant to be places of tranquil relaxation for patients. They had many windows that filled the area with natural light as well as areas where patients could sit and relax. These dayrooms faced the sunrise and were filled with light as the sun rose over the mountainside.

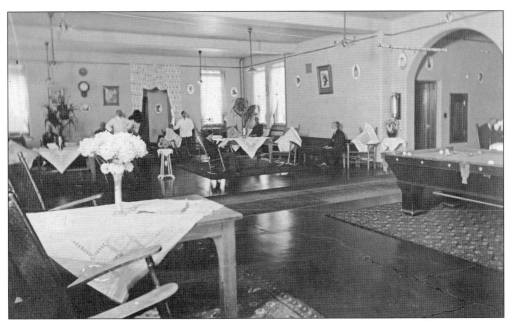

Each ward building featured these large dayrooms, which can be noted by the solarium-style architecture seen from the outside. The windows seen below illustrate these solarium formations. A typical dayroom consisted of many chairs, tables, pool tables, and pianos. It was the area where patients spent most of their day, socializing and interacting with each other. It was said that certain patients would play the most beautiful melodies each morning on the pianos in these rooms. The dayrooms were monitored by at least two nurses at all times. Hill Buildings 1 and 5 had three of these day rooms, whereas Hill Buildings 2 and 4 had two. (Both, courtesy of the Newark Public Library.)

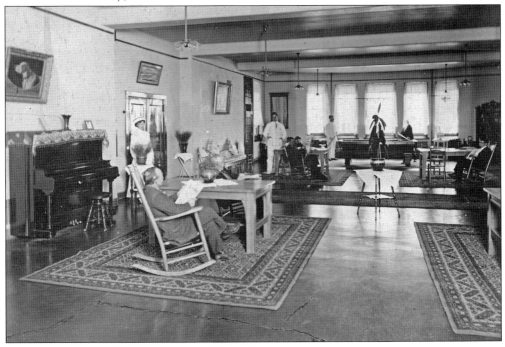

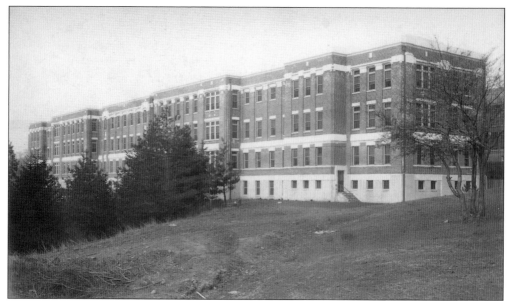

Building 11, the Reception Wards, was built in 1925 and was the largest building on campus after the Star Building. This four-story building, with three ward stories and a basement, housed Wards 53 through 58. It was built with a different architectural style than the Hill Buildings. New admissions were taken to the basement for processing. All medical issues were seen on the third floor. If patients had anything contagious, they were sent to the isolation hospital in Belleville. Disturbed patients were housed on the first floor of Reception. Depressed and suicidal patients were housed on the second floor. The building featured a state-of-the-art hydrotherapy room containing six tubs and a hose shower. Each ward also contained one tub for extended baths. The building was connected to Hill Building 3 via an elevated breezeway that was constructed during the modernizing renovations of the hospital.

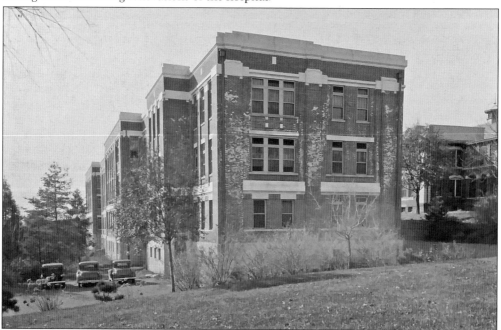

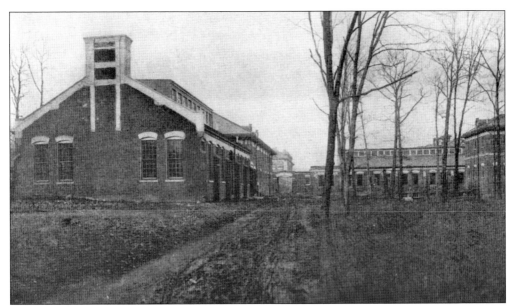

Building 8 was constructed with the Hill Buildings and served as the main kitchen for the entire hospital in the early years. Food was cooked in the kitchen and brought to each dining room. Hill Buildings 1 and 2 shared the female dining hall, Building 9. Hill Buildings 4 and 5 shared the male dining hall, Building 10. In 1919, ten kitchen messengers were employed to deliver food to the dining halls. (Courtesy of Robert L. Williams.)

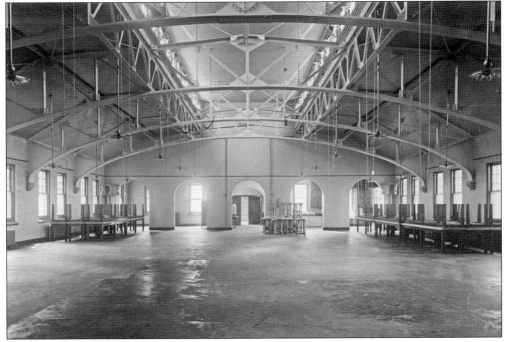

This 1936 photograph shows what the buildings looked like before and after each meal. Patients would sit down and be served by both kitchen staff and nurses. In 1960, drop ceilings were added, the male dining hall was redone with green tile walls, and the female dining hall was redone with pink tile walls. (Courtesy of the Newark Public Library.)

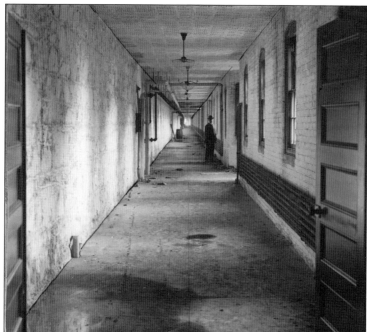

A long hallway extended from the back of the kitchen through the entire length of the complex. This hallway was used to deliver food to both dining halls, located at either end of the campus. The corridor was a third of a mile long, beginning at the kitchen, connecting to the female dining hall, Building 9, and ending at the male dining hall, Building 10. (Courtesy of the Newark Public Library.)

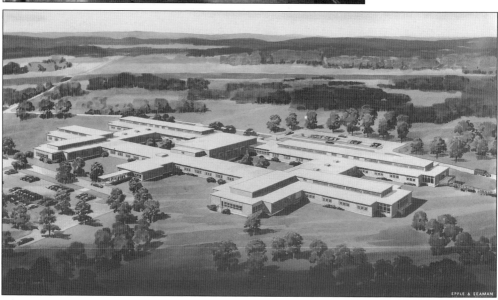

The Wright Pavilion was constructed in 1955 with a budget of $2,225,000, with $408,000 loaned by the state and county government. The building was dedicated to the treatment of elderly, mentally ill women. The building was referred to as a spread-plan layout, and everything was on one level. It was divided into three units, each with a 64-bed dormitory and a 48-bed dormitory. Basic health treatments were given inside this building, but for anything more than minor ailments, patients were sent to Building 11 for treatments. A kitchen and a cafeteria were inside the building, but meals were still supplied by the main kitchen, Building 8. The building remains today as a nursing home in Cedar Grove. The original frame of the building was kept, and the interior was redesigned to fit the needs of a modern nursing home. (Courtesy of the Newark Public Library.)

The Sunbeam

Volume 1, Number 4   July, August, September 1977 Edition

EMPTY AFTER EIGHTY ONE YEARS
STAR BUILDING TO BE REPLACED

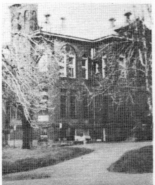

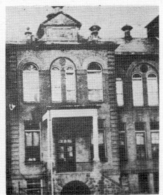

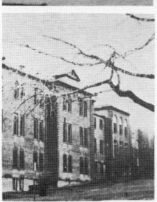

■ In 1896, the Essex County Board of Chosen Freeholders approved a contract for the purchase of 325 acres of farmland located in the Township of Verona, New Jersey, for the purpose of a new psychiatric hospital. The new site was located "Just Beyond the Brook", now known as the Peckman River, thus the name "Overbrook." This facility was to be primarily used for therapeutic treatment for patients in a farm atmosphere.

The first building at the hospital in Verona was called the Star Building; the reason for the name was because of the star-like configuration. The two-story building was fireproof and constructed of brick and iron. The first floor was adapted for use as day rooms, while the dormitories were located on the second floor. The basement area was used for the housing of employees, and administration personnel had apartments at the end of Wards 1 and 3.

During the summer of 1897, approximately one hundred patients were transferred to the new hospital from the South Orange Avenue Hospital for the Insane in Newark. Male patients were moved first to the hospital since it was felt that, while women were occupied with needlecraft to pass the hours, the men needed to be outdoors. A farm was promptly established, and it was expected that the harvest would be enough to supply the hospital. Also during 1897, two hundred and forty six patients were transferred to the building, and by 1907, the total population was four hundred and seventy eight patients, two hundred and eighteen females and two hundred and sixty males.

Patients were transported by trolley cars to the Erie Railroad Depot in Newark where a special train was provided. The Boys Brass Band from the Newark City Home met the train at Overbrook Station and played music as the patients disembarked and filed up the hill to the hospital.

The north side of Verona was separated from the south side and became the Township of Cedar Grove in 1908. Since that date the Star Building has had the reputation of being one of the oldest structures in Cedar Grove.

The South Orange Avenue facility

[Continued on Page Two]

In 1977, it was decided that the Star Building was to be demolished. An article in the July, August, September 1977 edition of the *Sunbeam* relayed the news. Although this was an internal publication, it was also available for purchase by the public.

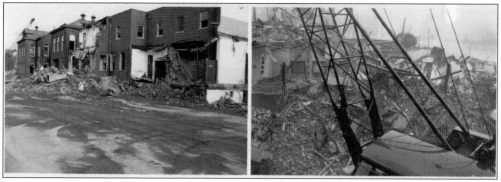

By the late 1970s, the Star Building had fallen into a state of disrepair. This was a very old building in need of major renovations. It was deemed more cost effective to demolish the Star Building than to try to maintain its condition.

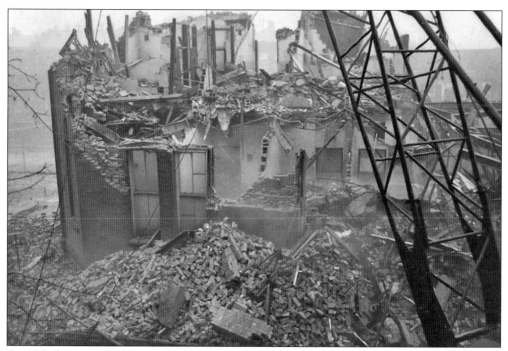

By 1979, the entire building had been demolished. After the Star Building disappeared, the rest of the main hospital ward buildings at Overbrook matched one another with the exception of the Reception Building. All buildings had the same redbrick exterior and windows with white brick and keystones.

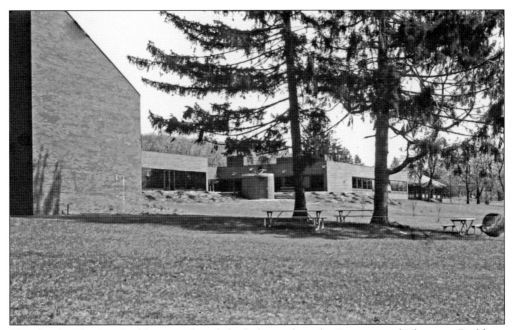

Shortly after the Star Building was demolished, the modern-day Recreational Therapies Building, Building 12, was constructed in its place. This was the activity center for the hospital. It featured a pool, gymnasium, bowling alley, and office-style sections. Outside of the building was a tennis court that patients and staff could use. (Courtesy of Justin Gurbisz.)

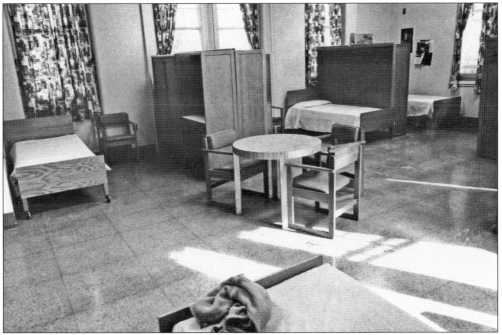

The inside of the Reception Building is seen in the 1970s, after the hospital's major modernization and renovation. A large portion of the building had been converted into mass patient rooms. A typical patient ward consists of 10–12 beds. Each bed came with a wardrobe for personal belongings that also doubled as a privacy barrier. (Courtesy of the Newark Public Library.)

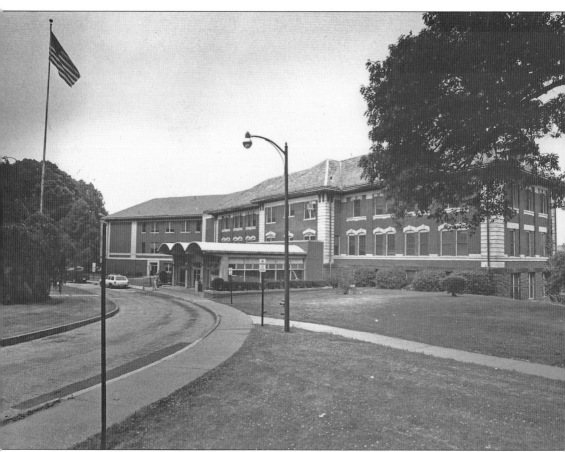

Beginning in 1960, major renovations were made to the Administration Building. The iconic original single-arch entryway structure became a three-arch entryway. This structure extended out from the original building and became the new main lobby for the hospital. An additional wing of offices was built and can be seen coming out from the left of the original structure. This addition can be noted by its different architecture around the windows, which featured whitish yellow ornamental brickwork with a center keystone. The inside of the building was also completely redone during this time. All of the elegant woodwork was removed, drop ceilings were installed, and the center staircase became the elevator shaft. The new Administration Building looked like a modern office building. (Courtesy of the Newark Public Library.)

Three

A City within Itself

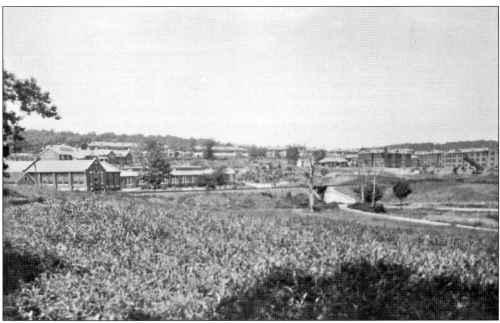

The Essex County Overbrook Hospital was a self-sustaining town within itself, able to operate without assistance from outside parties. Everything that a normal town would consist of—fire department, police department, power generating facilities, maintenance departments, farms, food storage, and more—was housed at Overbrook. The hospital had acres of farmland that extended out from the property up along Bradford Avenue in Cedar Grove. All food was raised or grown and prepared on site. Most of the furniture, mattresses, rugs, and window shades were made onsite either by patients or employees at the mechanics shop. For some time in the early 1900s, the hospital had its own postal code. Before the Caldwell Branch of the Erie Railroad was removed, the hospital had its own train station. Trains on that line also brought coal to the hospital's power plant, which was a short distance away from the main line. This plant ran power and steam to all the buildings on campus. Everything needed to keep the hospital functioning was on the grounds. (Courtesy of Robert L. Williams.)

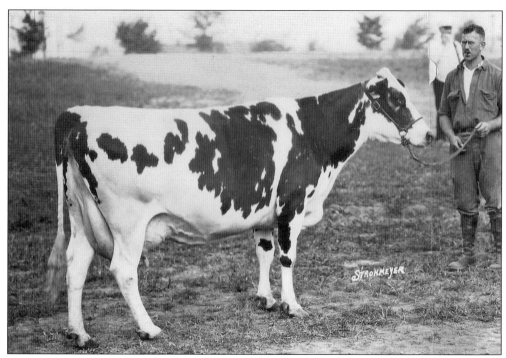

Overbrook raised cows for many purposes, mainly for meat and milk. This cow was an exception to that rule and lived at the hospital center as a world-famous prize holder. In 1926, the "Overbrook Prize Cow" won the grand championship at the Morristown Fair and third place at the Centennial World Fair in Philadelphia. (Courtesy of the Newark Public Library.)

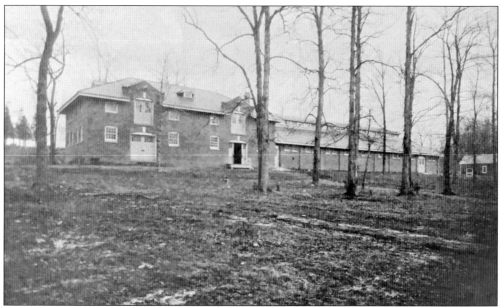

The Cow Barn is where all the cows at Overbrook were raised. The structure was in the agriculture section of the hospital campus by Bradford Avenue. Cows were housed, milked, and slaughtered for food here. This structure was proposed in the 1912 annual report.

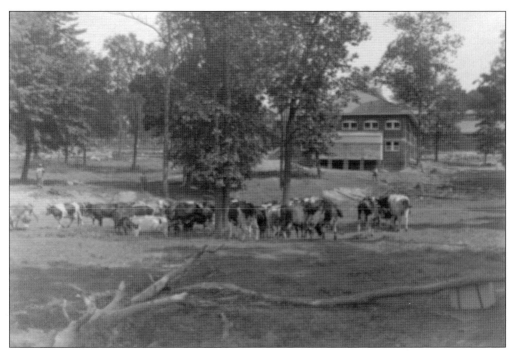

Most of the cattle at Overbrook roamed free across spacious land. The image was captured in 1914, during the phase when hospital agriculture was at one of its highest points. At Overbrook, a glass of milk was served every day with supper to promote strength and bone density in patients. Overbrook had the highest dairy-producing population in the United States, per the Holstein-Friesian Association of America.

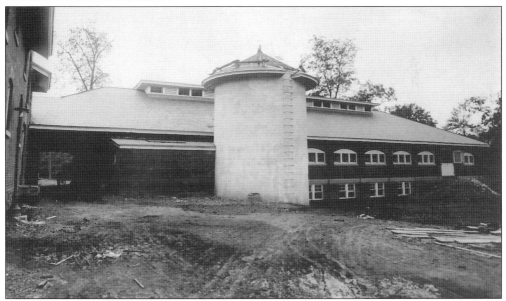

The Cow Barn is pictured after the addition of a silo. Overbrook had 190 cows and 10 bulls. In the early 1900s, this was the largest dairy herd in the Unites States. The herd produced around 1,140 quarts of milk per day for use by patients and staff. The herd also produced 1,500 pounds of manure per year to be taken to the Essex County Penitentiary. The dairy was disbanded in 1954.

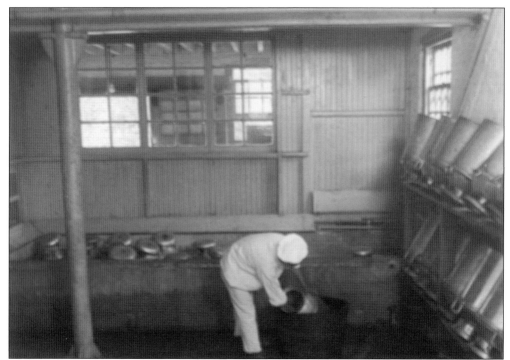

The milk harvested from the cows was stored in the large jugs seen above. The jugs were then transferred from the Cow Barn to the Storehouse for proper storage. Above, an employee places the pails of milk in the Storehouse in 1914. The cooling system was similar to that of a root cellar, where a section was dug out underground for natural refrigeration.

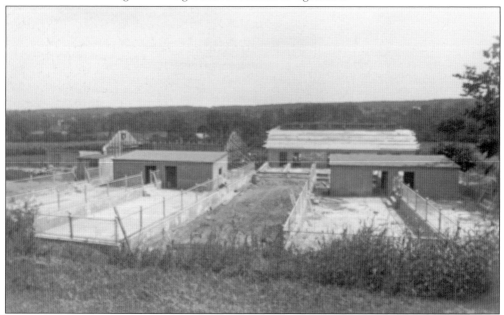

Pigs were also raised in Overbrook's agricultural areas to be slaughtered for food for the hospital patients and staff. Pigpens and the pig yard were established in 1898 in the farming area along Bradford Avenue. On average, Overbrook kept 353 pigs per year.

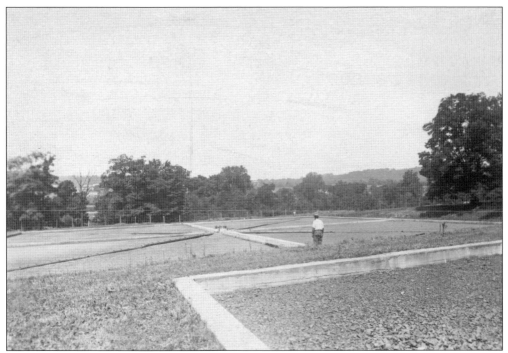

The farmland dedicated for Overbrook was established in 1898. All fruits and vegetables consumed by patients at Overbrook were grown on site. The farmland was outfitted with a system of pipes to irrigate the crops. The main well and pumping station for watering the crops were located on the east side of the railroad tracks. A half-acre pond with an icehouse and a water treatment plant were also located in this area.

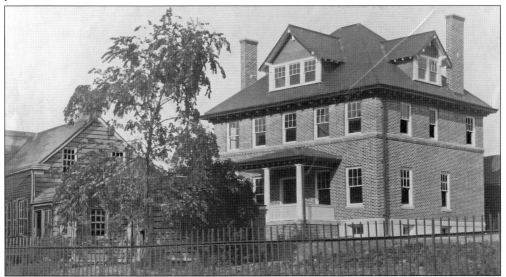

This photograph, taken in June 1920, shows both the farmers' old residence and the new farmers' cottage at Overbrook. The house to the left was the original farmhouse for the farmer and his family. This house, 106 years old by 1917, was falling apart by 1912, and a new structure was called for. The cottage on the right was the newer farmhouse, used after the original was abandoned. The new farmers' cottage cost $50,000 to construct. (Courtesy of the Newark Public Library.)

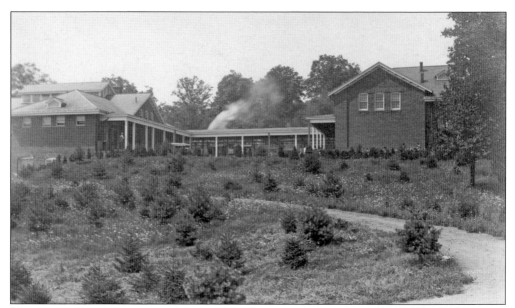

The Storehouse was an essential structure in the functionality of Overbrook. The building was used to store food and featured old-style cold-box structures dug into the ground to keep perishable foods cold, along with meat hanging racks behind the building. The railroad tracks went alongside the building to deliver shipments of food and resources. The building was demolished in two phases. The last remains of the building were demolished around 2010.

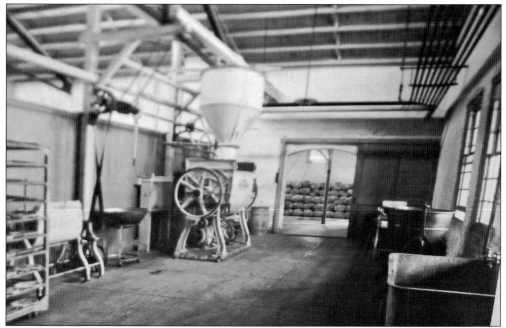

The bakery was a separate building next to the Storehouse. In 1960, the department was run by Ernest A. Dangel and his crew. They baked around 2,200 loaves of bread a day, 614,893 for the year. The loaves were used at Overbrook and also sent to the penitentiary, sanatorium, and hospital in Belleville. In 1960, Overbrook used half a million pounds of flour and four and a half tons of yeast. (Courtesy of Robert L. Williams.)

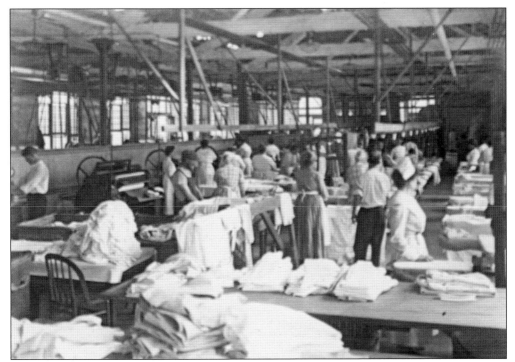

The laundry building was part of the maintenance group in close proximity to the powerhouse. All the clothing, bedsheets, rugs, carpets, and any other linen or fabric was cleaned in this building. Hospital staff made an effort to always keep soiled linens separate from washed material in effort to keep everything sanitary.

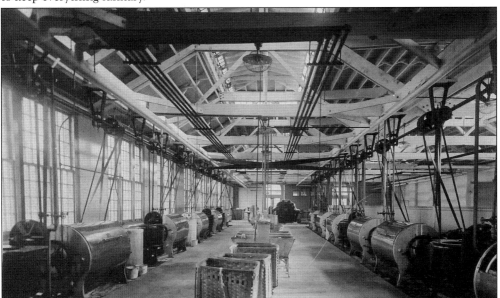

In 1960, the laundry building processed 5,395,214 pounds of linen and clothes. It also dyed 13,800 pounds of new linen for the wards. The laundry was also in charge of pressing clothing for patients and pressed 51,272 patients' shirts in 1960. It also dry-cleaned 8,500 clothing articles in 1960. This photograph was taken in the early 1900s. (Courtesy of the Newark Public Library.)

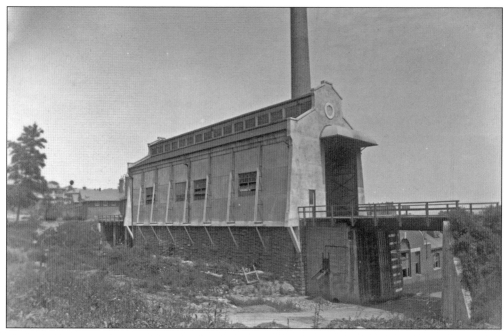

Overbrook's powerhouse initially consisted of two main structures. The first was the coal tipple. This 1914 photograph shows the coal-receiving tipple of the powerhouse. Coal was delivered by trains coming from an offshoot of the Caldwell branch of the Erie Railroad that extended onto campus. The railroad tracks can clearly be seen going into the structure.

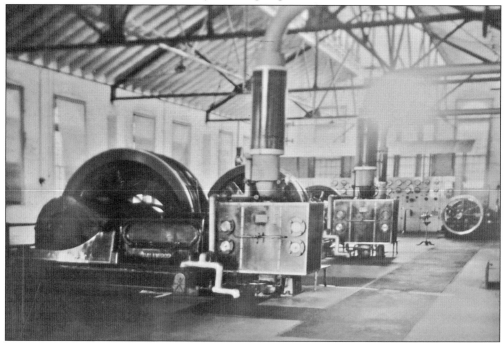

The other original structure at Overbrook's powerhouse was the generating room. Here, power and steam were made and sent into the buildings through pipes in underground tunnels. In 1960, the powerhouse produced 445 million pounds of steam. (Courtesy of Robert L. Williams.)

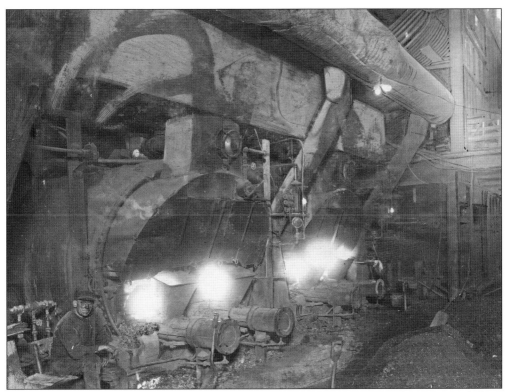

The old boiler room shows two of the original boilers in operation. These did not provide heat to the main institution. They were used to provide power for electricity and laundry services. The buildings of the main institution relied on pot stoves, open fires, and oil heaters for heating. This information is cited directly from Overbrook's annual report books. (Courtesy of the Newark Public Library.)

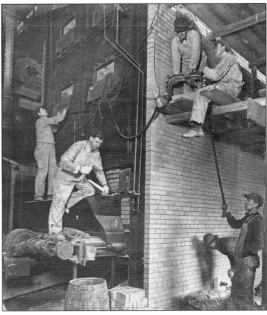

In 1917, the powerhouse received new boilers following an earlier boiler malfunction. By adding more machinery, the main institutional buildings could rely on heat from the powerhouse instead of using their own means of heating. In 1960, the hospital produced 7,219,000 kilowatt hours of electricity. (Courtesy of the Newark Public Library.)

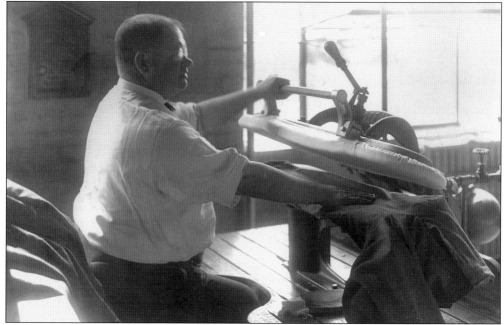

In addition to generating its own power and food sources, the hospital also manufactured and maintained essential everyday items used in the complex. Seen here is the process in which county employees pressed recently made clothes. Patients would also handcraft clothing to be distributed throughout the hospital to be used by other patients.

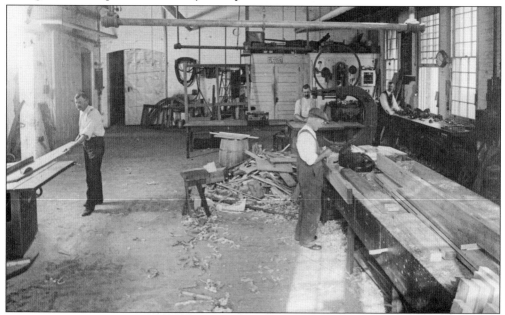

An interior view shows the mechanics shop as seen in chapter 2. Workers are building materials for use in the hospital center. This was the only building on Overbrook's campus to be used and maintained by Essex County after the hospital's abandonment. The turn-of-the-century brick building was completely remodeled with stucco in 2013 and, unfortunately, abandoned in 2016 and demolished in 2017.

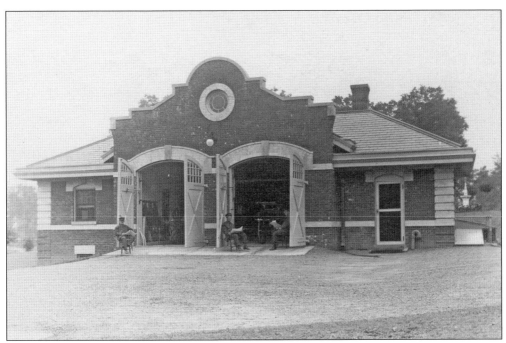

The hospital's original firehouse is seen in 1914. This building was right off Fairview Avenue on the same eastern side of campus as the main hospital. The firehouse was fully equipped to deal with any fire hazard that might occur on campus. The fire crew was a smaller staff and consisted of one patient volunteer in 1912. Original firefighting equipment can be seen below. In 1913, it was suggested that a new firehouse be constructed to accommodate more modern fire engines and a growing staff.

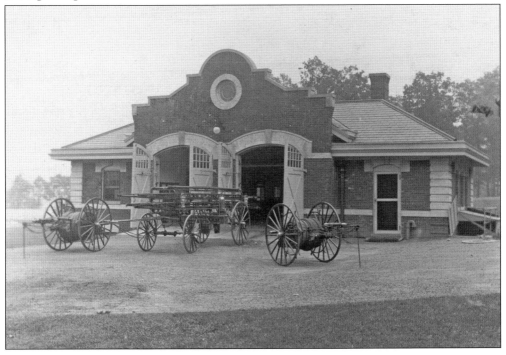

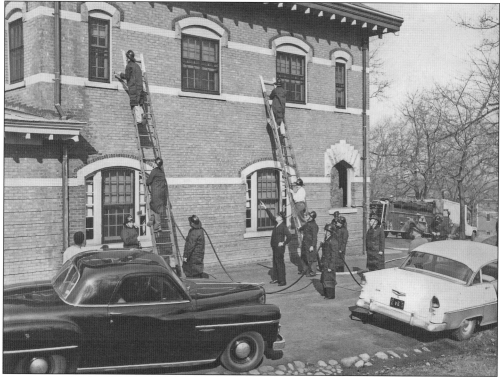

The new firehouse, which was constructed in 1915, was on the west side of Fairview Avenue. The building had two garages and featured living quarters for firehouse personnel. By 1917, the structure was in full use and was just awaiting the completion of the living quarters.

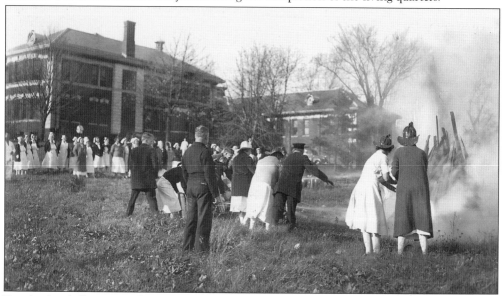

Regular fire drills were performed at Overbrook by starting a small controlled fire outdoors on the grounds of the hospital. Fire personnel supervised and taught the proper procedures for putting out the controlled blazes. Staff members were required to both observe and participate in the drills, as seen in the photograph above.

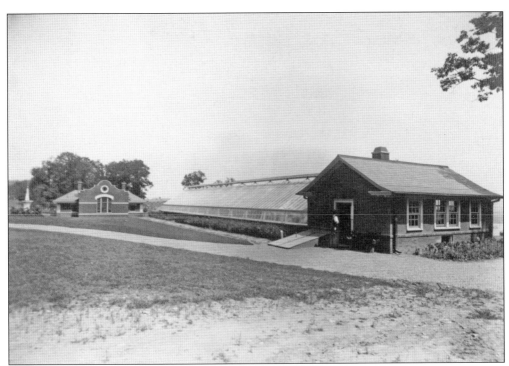

The greenhouse at Overbrook was next to the original firehouse on the east side of Fairview Avenue, as this 1914 photograph shows. The greenhouse keeper was responsible for growing the ornamental flowers that were placed throughout the hospital. Fresh flowers were placed in all the ward dayrooms, connector hallways, and dining rooms.

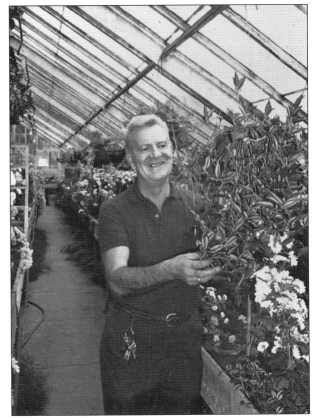

The greenhouse keeper played a key role in creating an atmosphere at the hospital. Here he is showing off the interior of the greenhouse and the plants and flowers used to decorate the hospital buildings. The greenhouse keeper lived in a small two-story home next to the greenhouse.

Overbrook Jottings

Published Monthly by Essex County Hospital

Cedar Grove, N. J., July, 1929

Price, 10c. Per Copy
Subscription: $1.00 Per Year

OBSERVES ...ENDENCE DAY

...rved Independence ...honored manner on ...ightful program of ...musical numbers ...g was given in the ...ing was led by the ...The program was ...p singing of "The ...nner" and "Amer- ..."The Old Flag ...tho Ground," was ...the patients. Miss ...sang two solos, ...to Old Virginny" ...he Beautiful." A ...given to dancing, ...g being furnished ...orchestra. ...ram in the Audi- ...its marched to the ...the ball game be- ...and the Pitkin ...es' Band led the ...he game the ever ...was dispensed, and ...were given by the

COW HANGS ...THER RECORD

...y continues to dis- ...l individuals of the ...apple records. The ...Speckled Bess, a ...d at Overbrook, and

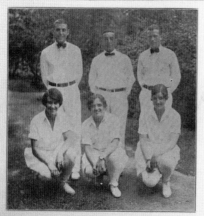

STAFF OF PHYSICAL EDUCATION DEPARTMENT
TOP ROW, LEFT TO RIGHT: ALBERT CIANIRELLI, MORRIS SACHS, PHYSICAL DIRECTOR; WILLIAM McGARR; BOTTOM ROW: ELEANOR B. MAHLER, ESTHER KUSNER AND MARY LOU LILLIS.

Sixteenth Annual Field Day of Best on Record; Hundreds of Visitors Present

1000 Pullets Purchased.

Overbrook's hennery has just received shipment of 1,000 two-months old pullets from the Wene Chick Farms of Vineland, N. J. From the looks of the pullets there will be many a hard-boiled egg about Overbrook next winter, according to Supervisor George Taylor, who has the management of the hennery.

INTERESTING PAPERS AT ASSOCIATION MEET

Dr. Payne, Miss Morris and Miss Lunger attended the National Occupational Therapy Association at Atlantic City last month, and report a most interesting meeting. Our department had exhibits of its producets.

There were several hundred delegates at the meeting, and exhibits were there from institutions all over the country. One of the most interesting features was an exhibit of "undirected activities." In this exhibit were original creations of school workers, which had been done without direction at all of school instructors, and included metal work and the several crafts. It was presented as an avenue of approach and study of the mental content of the worker. Many interesting papers were on the program.

After a few weeks at 685 Summer Avenue, Newark, the Occupational Therapy department moved its sales-

RECREATIONAL CLUB ENJOYS DOG ROAST

On Tuesday evening, July 9, about twenty-five members of the club and their friends adjourned to Lake Apache where all enjoyed a very refreshing swim, after which they roasted hot dogs and marshmallows. Although the road was rather rough and muddy they finally succeeded in reaching their destination.

After an hour's swim came the luncheon of hot-dogs, lettuce, tomatoes, relish and soda. True to Indian style, all sat around the fire and sang songs, which were interrupted by several Apache dances given by two male members of the party. Aside from the fact that the time went too quickly, everyone had a wonderful time, returning home tired but happy. From comments that have been heard throughout the hospital, everyone is looking forward to another good time shortly.

DOCTOR HATCHER AND FAMILY ON VACATION

Dr. George A. Hatcher and family left by motor the morning of July 4 for their vacation on their farm in Williamson County, Tennessee. They went by Niagara Falls, and from Buffalo they went to Cleveland by boat. Cards posted in Cleveland the morning of July 5 were received

---

The Sunbeam

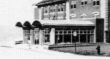

Volume 1, Number 1   July, August, September Issues 1974   Carol Ann Gartner, Editor

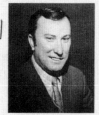

MICHAEL P. DUFFY

- Michael P. Duffy, presently serving as Superintendent of both the Essex County Hospital Center in Cedar Grove and the Essex County Geriatrics Center in Belleville, is a resident of Maplewood, New Jersey. He graduated from Seton Hall Preparatory School in South Orange and he received a B.A. degree in Education from Newark State College in Union. In his present fulfillment as Superintendent at the Essex County Hospital Center and the Essex County Geriatrics Center, he is the direct administrator of business coordination at both hospitals.
Mr. Duffy's background before coming to the Hospital Center is varied and diversified. He served at the Essex County Geriatrics Center as Secretary to the Superintendent, which entailed administering to the needs of 450 em-
[continued on page two]

EDITORIAL NOTE

■ This is the first issue of our newsletter since the appointment of the new Superintendent and Medical Director.
We will give a brief biographical outline of their careers to date in hopes that you will get to know them. In future issues of this newsletter, we will be featuring other personalities at the Hospital Center. C.R.

~

[From left to right] Standing: Steve Racin, Roosevelt Perkins, Dominick Giantomase, Roderick Andress. Seated: Eleanor Harin, Frank Antonacci and Florence Brovette.

X-RAY DEPARTMENT

CONTEST WINNER

■ The contest to name our Newsletter was won by the X-Ray Department, with a winning entry "The Sunbeam." Many names were submitted and choosing the title was
[continued on page two]

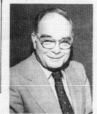

FELIX A. UCKO, M.D.

■ Dr. Felix A. Ucko, the Essex County Hospital Center's newly appointed Medical Director, has had a long career in the psychiatric and medical fields.
Born in New York City, Dr. Ucko graduated from medical school in Frankfurt, Germany. He served as an assistant in Pharmacology in Biefeld, Germany and as an assistant in Internal Medicine at the University of Frankfurt, Germany. Dr. Ucko completed his internship in New York City Hospital, Welfare Island, New York. After a two year rotating residency at Irvington General Hospital, he came to the Essex County Hospital Center to serve his psychiatric residency.
During the Korean conflict, he
[continued on page two]

The Essex County Overbrook Hospital had its own printing press that put out multiple publications within the hospital. One popular publication was the monthly *Overbrook Jottings*, which covered various topics on staff, events, and patients. This 1929 copy discusses everything from the physical education staff to the family vacations of prominent doctors in the hospital.

The *Sunbeam* was a quarterly publication put out by Overbrook. This July, August, September 1974 edition gives an example of the work. The newsletter opens with recognition of both the newly appointed superintendent and the medical director. This was similar to the *Overbrook Jottings*, in that it covered a wide array of topics involving the hospital center.

Four

STAFF AND PATIENTS

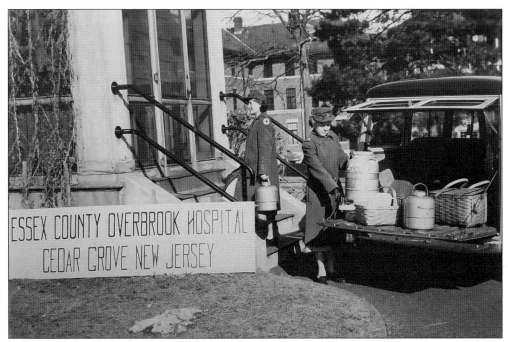

Workers are greeted by a handmade sign as they enter a screened-in porch with a delivery of goods from nearby Montclair. Overbrook had an outpatient facility in Montclair that was founded in 1960. Many local communities frequently traded or donated goods to the hospital center, as they shared a sense of compassion for patients at Overbrook. (Courtesy of Newark Public Library.)

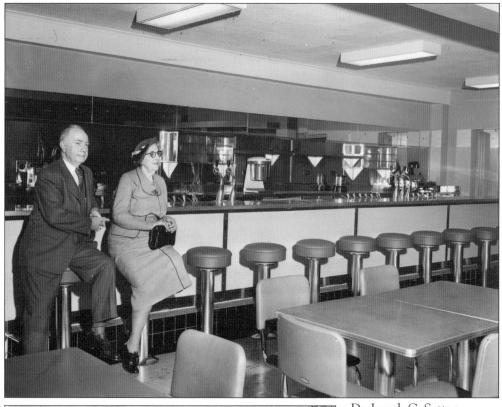

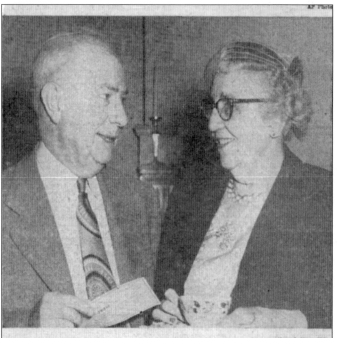

Dr. Joseph G. Sutton, medical director, poses for photographs in a café-type seating area with Essex freeholder Eliza G. Wright. Mrs. Wright was the Essex freeholder director from 1956 to 1958. She was succeeded in 1959 and 1960 by Jean Moss. (Courtesy of Newark Public Library.)

As documented in this excerpt from the *Newark News*, Dr. Joseph Sutton led a collection fund among the employees at the hospital to build a nondenominational chapel. A total of $500 was allotted, which was handed over to freeholder director Eliza G. Wright. The chapel was located in the service building, Building 7.

Newark News Photo

FOR CHAPEL—Mrs. Eliza G. Wright, Essex Freeholders director, receives $500 check yesterday from Dr. Joseph G. Sutton, medical director of Overbrook Hospital, Cedar Grove. Hospital staff gave money for fund for interdenominational chapel at hospital.

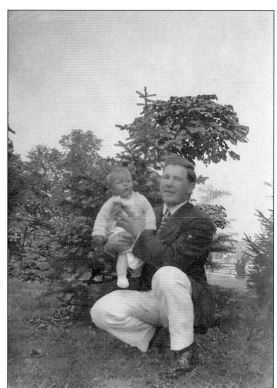

Dr. Guy Payne Jr. was born in Cedar Grove in 1907 and served as medical superintendent of Overbrook Hospital. His father, Guy Payne Sr., was also a physician. He served as medical director from 1910 to 1947, with a leave of absence during his time serving in World War I. Dr. Payne Jr. attended elementary school at nearby Montclair Academy and graduated from Union College in Schenectady, New York, in June 1928. He passed away on April 23, 1978, at his home in Hyde Park, Vermont.

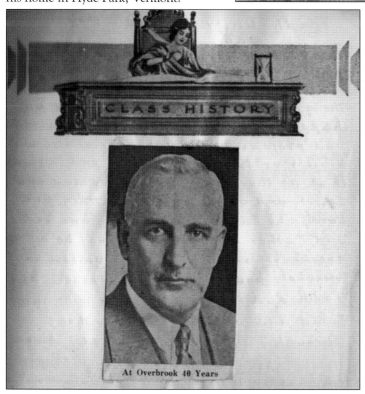

CLASS HISTORY

At Overbrook 40 Years

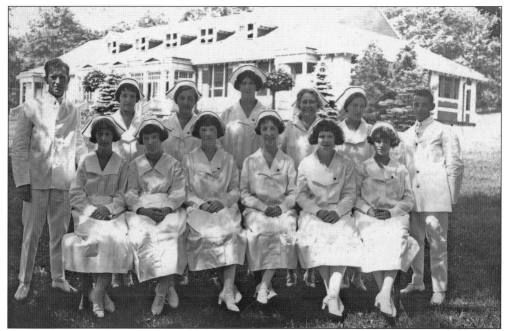

In this 1924 photograph, members of the x-ray department line up for group portrait. At this time, this technology was still relatively new. Most of the x-rays were performed to screen patients' lungs for the ever-growing threat of tuberculosis, and some patients were then treated at the nearby Essex Mountain Sanatorium.

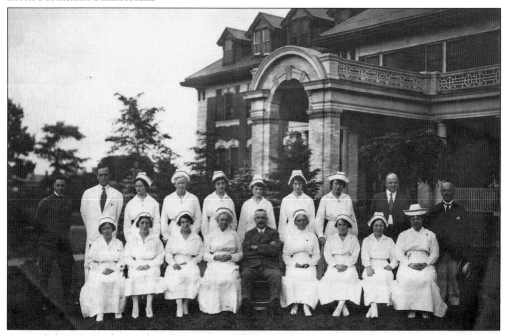

Around the 1920s, doctoral and nursing staff pose in front of the Administration Building on Fairview Avenue. The building had several changes in appearance over the years, including modern additions and the use of an enclosed glass hallway as an entrance in later years, before being demolished in 2016.

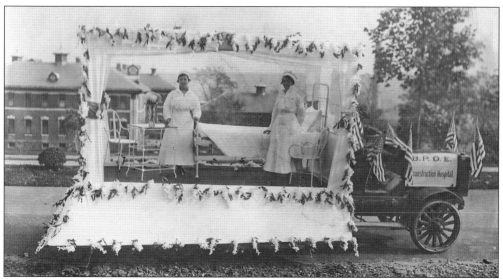

This undated photograph features a float with nursing staff aboard to promote the hospital, as sponsored for a holiday parade by the Benevolent and Protective Order of Elks, also known as the Elks Lodge. Staff members of the hospital took great pride in their work and frequently appeared in community events.

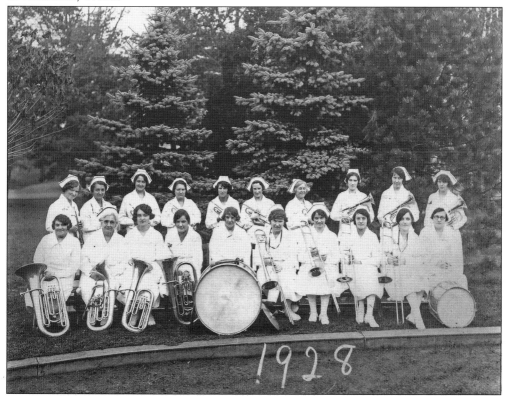

Taken in 1928, this photograph shows one of the many ways that even the hospital staff received enrichment. A number of bands were formed that often performed for patients or nearby residents on the grounds of the hospital. This particular photograph shows the female nurses' band.

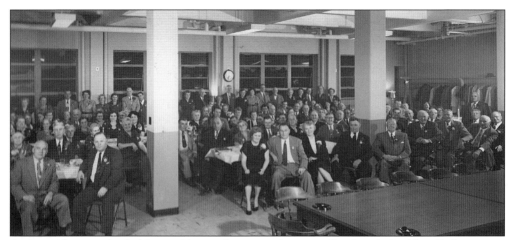

A group of county freeholders and hospital personnel meet at Overbrook. Building 7, the service building, housed a conference room on its second floor. This building was constructed in 1951 and became a spot for staff and county members to hold meetings. The building also housed the chapel and libraries.

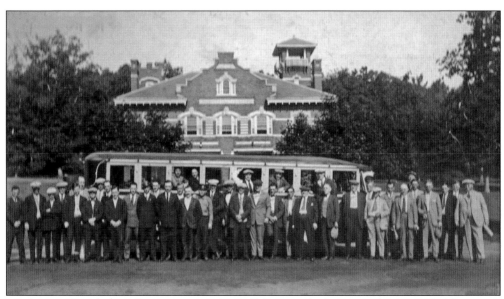

Faculty members line up for an outing in front of the 1915 firehouse on the west side of Fairview Avenue. This building was demolished in late 2015, leaving only the smaller building directly across the street.

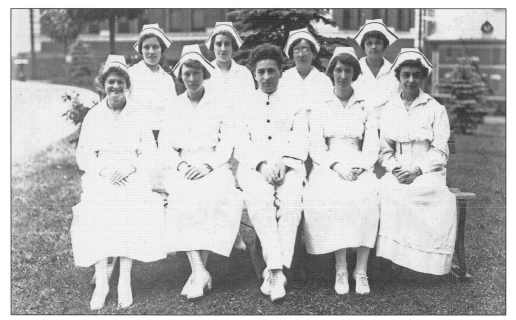

Nursing staff pose on the front lawn of the Administration Building in the mid-1920s. Their uniforms are typical of that time period, including white stockings and high-heeled shoes for the women and button-up collared shirts for the men. Nursing crews were highly skilled and aimed to get the patients discharged from the hospital and in a better state of mind.

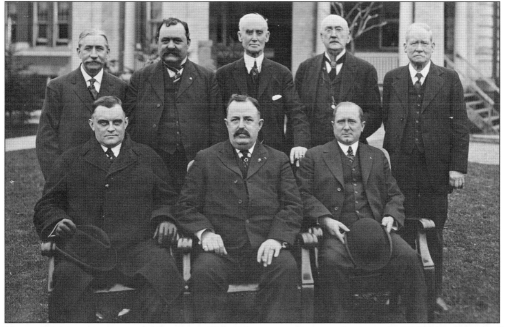

Hospital administrative and doctoral staff pose for a typical group photograph near the entrance of the Administrative Building. Group photographs were common in the early years of the hospital and were aimed to give representation to the different groups of staff members working at the hospital center. Employees such as doctors, nurses, maintenance crews, and financial staff would all have group photographs taken.

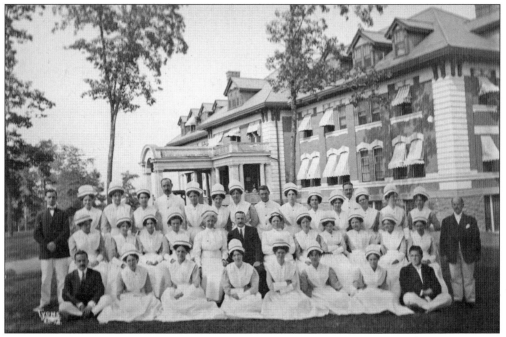

Support staff and faculty members line up on the front lawn of the hospital near the main entrance. Nurses, both male and female, are featured in the photograph. The year 1957 was one of the best for staffing at Overbrook. The staff went from 975 to 1,049 total employees working at the hospital center.

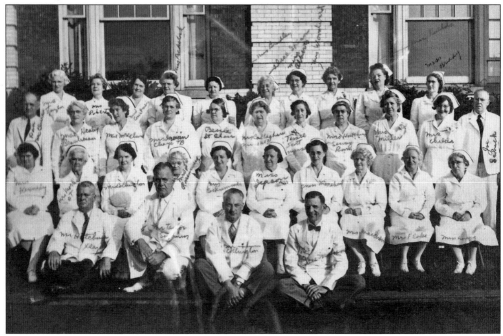

Hospital caregivers pose for a slightly less formal photograph during the 1920s. Their names and corresponding titles are written in cursive over the original photograph, with such examples as "Mr. Hutchinson" from x-ray and "Mrs. Callagham" from Ward 13.

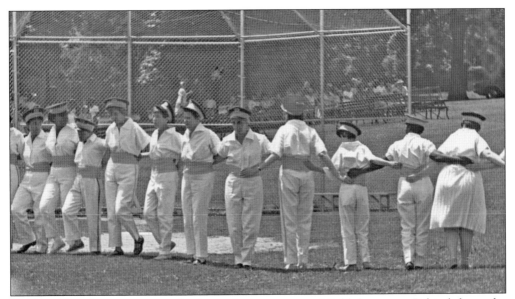

Staff members line up as part of a dance during an annual field day event. Behind them, the baseball fence and home base can be seen. In 1911, it was proposed that the fence be built along with a grandstand for seating. Before this, patients and staff sat on the grass along the hill overlooking the field.

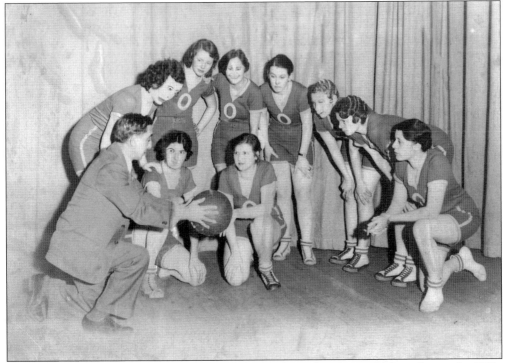

Women basketball players can be seen wearing official Overbrook team T-shirts during the 1931–1932 season. The basketball team consisted of female employees of the hospital. Staff members participated in many team sports against other local communities while working at the hospital. They also competed against other hospitals that had their own teams.

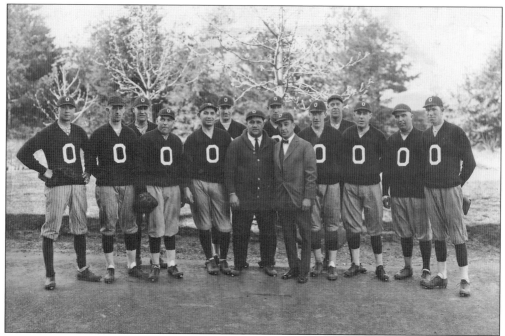

Male baseball players pose in their official Overbrook team uniforms in this 1930s photograph. The coaches can be distinguished from the players in this photograph. Both coaches and all team players were staff members at Overbrook.

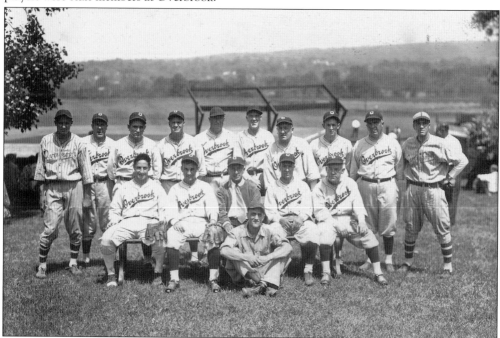

The men's staff baseball team is shown on the field behind the ward buildings in 1936. The baseball team competed against local communities and teams. Many of the employees who participated in Overbrook's baseball team were highly skilled. The area where the baseball field was is now part of Cedar Grove Park and Community Center.

During a tour of the hospital grounds in the 1960s, this photograph documents the ground-level connector walkway from the rear of Building 3 to Building 11. This is an outdoor set of stairs that connects the two buildings. Initially, there was a walkway between Building 3 and the Star Building. This was renovated into the outdoor staircase when Building 11 was constructed in 1925. (Courtesy of Newark Public Library.)

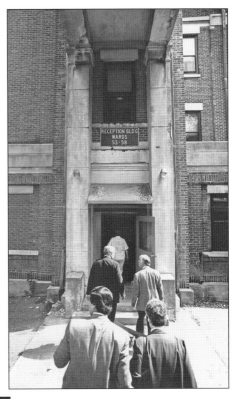

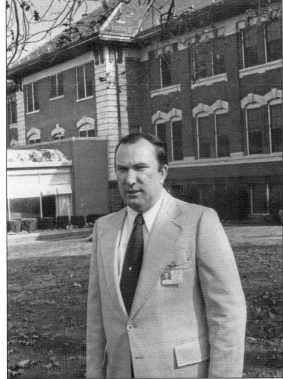

In this 1970s photograph, hospital superintendent Michael P. Duffy is visible on the front lawn of the hospital. He was also superintendent of the Essex County Isolation Hospital in Belleville through the 1960s and 1970s. (Courtesy of Newark Public Library.)

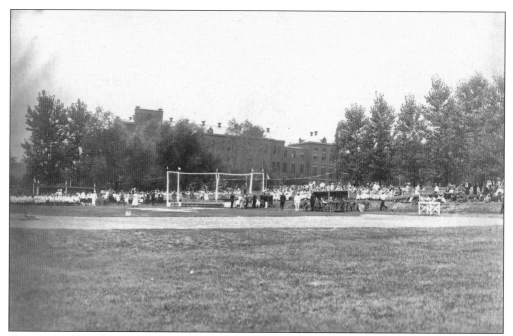

Patients, staff, and community members lined the fields behind the Star Building for numerous festivities. This photograph depicts the Essex County Hospital Center's annual field day event. The first field day was held in 1911, and it soon became a staple of the hospital's history. Both patients and staff participated in various events during the field day.

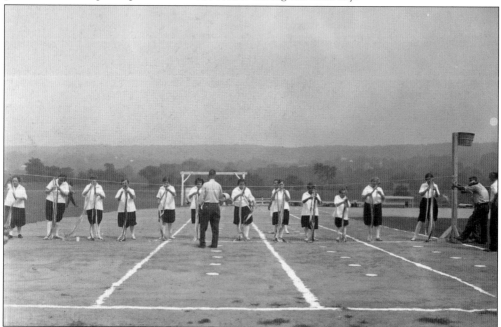

In this photograph, dated July 22, 1936, patients and staff can be seen participating in group activities on the rear athletic fields. This served as a form of recreational therapy that lasted until the final days of the hospital. The recreational therapy department was run by an average of five staff members.

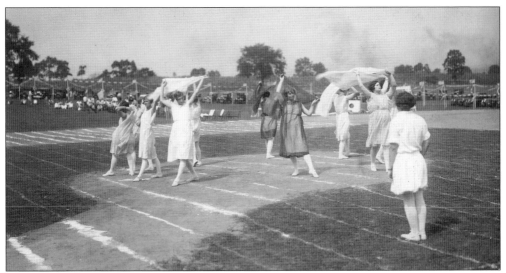

Women are seen performing as part of festivities. The hospital complex was home to its own tailor shop, so the outfits and costumes featured in many of these photographs were often created by patients and staff as part of occupational therapies.

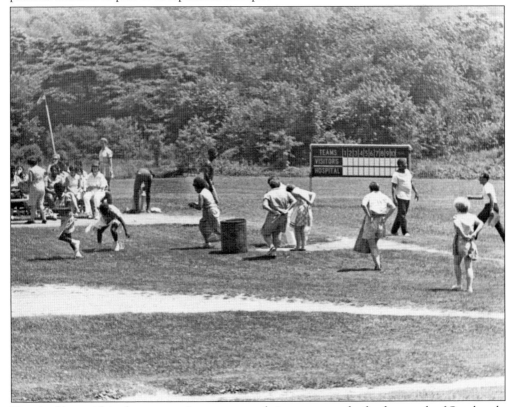

Teambuilding within the community was extremely important to the fundamentals of Overbrook. In this c. 1930s photograph, a scoreboard can be seen in the background for "Visitors" versus "Hospital." Onlookers consisting of staff and neighbors are seated on the bleachers and grandstand that were constructed in 1911.

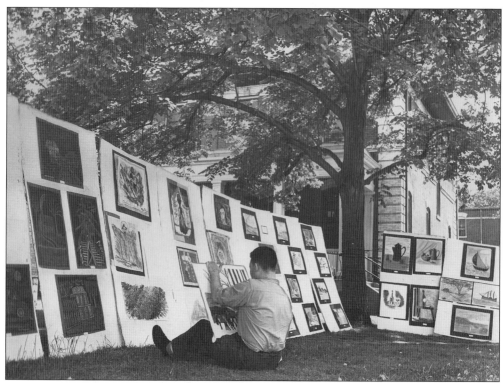

In this undated photograph, an artist sets up a display outside of an iconic Hill Ward Building with a view of the kitchen hallway in the background. Staff, patients, and members of the community were encouraged to participate in social activities at the hospital. It was common to host social gatherings on the lawns during the summer. (Courtesy of Newark Public Library.)

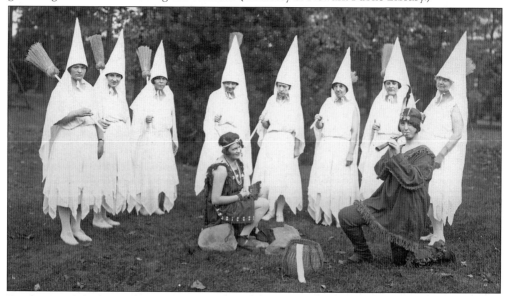

Employees of the hospital participate in a program titled "Hallowe'en Witches, Indian Flapper and Young Brave" during October 1927, as photographed by R.T. Elson. The costumes and props featured in the performance were made onsite by patients as part of occupational therapies.

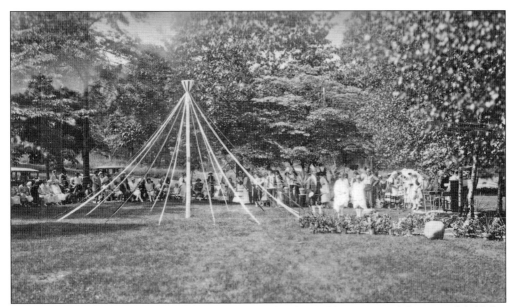

Staff and patients enjoy an outdoor festival in 1936. This field was part of the annual field day and served as another area for plays to be held. The bandstand was mostly reserved for outdoor musical performances. This small open field bordering the woods behind the hospital was used as an outdoor auditorium.

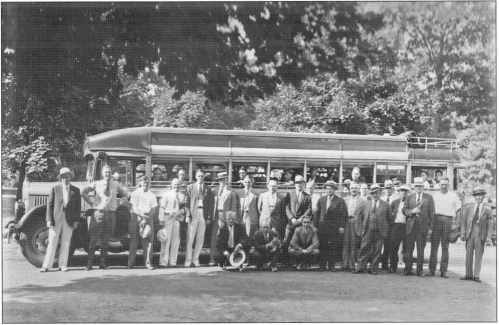

Staff members prepare to board a chartered bus to visit Manhattan Beach in 1934 with a few select patients, including Red Taylor, invited to join them. Several names of participants are listed on an attached sheet of paper, including Charlie Childs, Frank Conway, Paul Jennings, Eddy Hector, Tom Pickstock, and "Smitty" the electrician. Nonviolent patients who did not pose a threat were frequently allowed to take daytrips, so long as they returned by the evening and complied with their medical treatments.

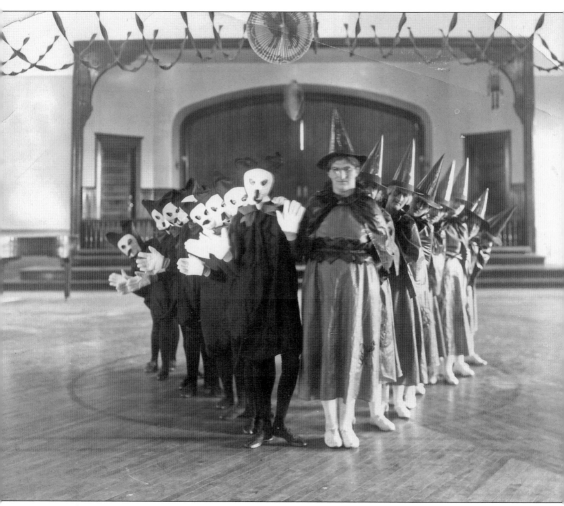

Faculty members put on a Halloween performance to entertain coworkers as well as patients of Overbrook. The recreational therapy department at Overbrook was responsible for sponsoring these plays. It sponsored the Halloween performance, a performance of Washington crossing the Delaware, Christmas entertainment, the annual field day, and other dances for Overbrook's patients and staff. Plays were put on throughout the year in Assembly Hall, the auditorium.

This promotional flyer was circulated for a performance titled *Life in a Sanitarium*, dated April 18, 1912. Patients were given many forms of activities to express themselves and entertain their cohabitants. It is important to note the difference between a sanitarium and a sanatorium. With the close proximity to the Essex Mountain Sanatorium, the two were often confused. However, the former refers to a mental institution, while the latter is related to the treatment of tuberculosis.

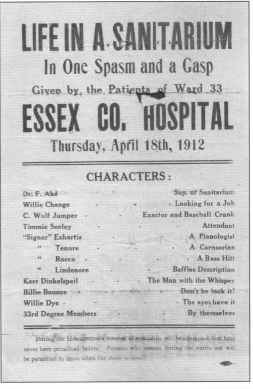

LIFE IN A·SANITARIUM
In One Spasm and a Gasp
Given by the Patients of Ward 33
ESSEX CO. HOSPITAL
Thursday, April 18th, 1912

CHARACTERS :

Dr. F. Ake	Sup. of Sanitarium
Willie Change	Looking for a Job
C. Wolf Jumper	Exactor and Baseball Crank
Timmie Seeley	Attendant
"Signor" Exhartis	A Pianologist
" Tenore	A Carnsorian
" Rocco	A Bass Hitt
" Lindenore	Baffles Description
Kerr Dinkelspeil	The Man with the Whisper
Billie Bounce	Don't he look it?
Willie Dye	The ayes have it
33rd Degree Members	By themselves

During the Indescretion a number of specialties will be attempted that have never been permitted before. Patients who remain during the entire act will be permitted to leave when the show is over.

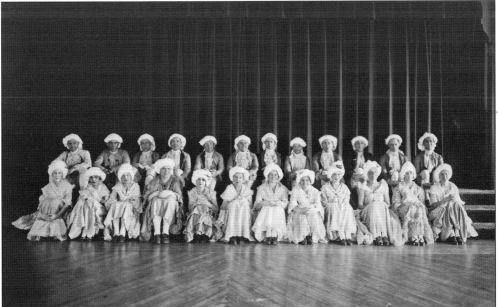

On March 2, 1939, both male and female patients dress in Colonial attire to present a play in the hospital's auditorium. During these times, people were committed to mental institutions for a variety of reasons. Many patients were otherwise unaffected by their diagnoses, while some were held on the basis of intellectual disability only. Under the watchful eye of the faculty, thousands of people at Overbrook successfully participated in group programs such as this.

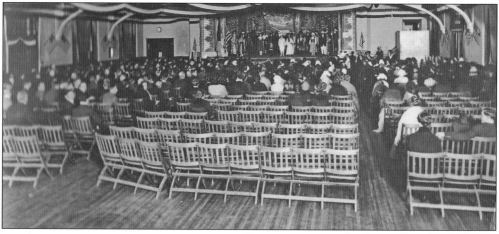

Patients present a play during Fourth of July celebrations in the 1930s as hospital staff and community members look on. The architecture of the auditorium is similar to that of the dining halls on the main hospital campus. The main difference that can be noted is the stage and doorways to its left and right.

Three-day Overbrook Fair And Halloween Dance on Tap

Patients and personnel at Essex County Overbrook Hospital, Cedar Grove, were busy this week completing arrangements for the hospital's fifty-third annual Fall fair and annual Halloween dance. A variety of articles made by patients during the past year in the Occupational Therapy Department will be offered for sale at the fair which is being held today, tomorrow and Saturday. The articles include rugs, linens, lamps, handcraft, etc. The fair is being sponsored by the department. Clive Krygar Jr. of Orange, director of the department, recently received his master's degree in education from Rutgers University.

The purpose of the department's program, according to Krygar, is to provide an opportunity for the patients to do things with other people in an environment free of pressure in order that they may meet their problems successively on a small scale and begin overcoming them.

Dr. Henry A. Davidson, hospital superintendent and medical director, said the medical-psychological aspects of occupational therapy are among the hospital's most important functions.

A young Brazilian Nisei girl, Miss Masako Ito, and Milton Crawley, physical therapy director, will lead the grand march at the Halloween dance tonight at the hospital's gaily decorated Guy Payne auditorium.

Miss Ito, a music intern in the Music and Creative Arts Department, is a native of Sao Paulo, Brazil. She came to the United States six years a to continue her studies tow a career as a concert pia Several months ago she doned her career to c Overbrook Hospital t music therapy.

More than 200 pat attend the dance in some of them made tients and others d civic organizations.

and hospital officials and personnel and relatives and friends of patients also will attend.

The program will include novelty dances, a waltz contest, a skit performed by patients and a salute to the women of the geriatric section. Music will be provided by the patients' orchestra. Refreshments will be served at the dance and in the hospital wards to patients unable to attend the dance.

This newspaper clipping from the *Verona–Cedar Grove Times* describes a three-day event at the hospital in October 1963. The programs included dance festivities, skits, and orchestras presented by the patients as part of the Music and Creative Arts Department. Community members were also presented with the opportunity to purchase handmade goods produced by Overbrook.

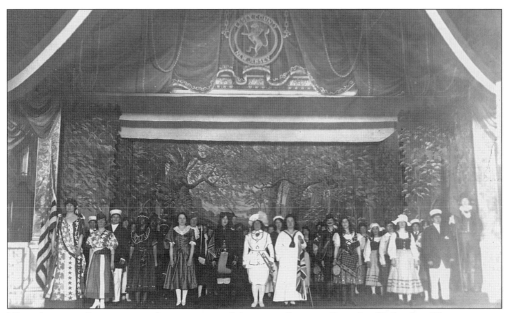

This photograph presents a close-up view of the stage during a Fourth of July play. The attention to detail can be vividly noted, with hand-painted backgrounds, intricate outfits, decorations hung from the ceiling rafters, and the Essex County logo.

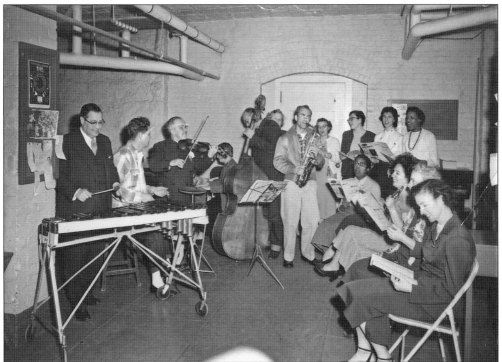

The Music and Creative Arts Department, located in the basement of Building 3, was home to Overbrook's very own patient orchestra. A variety of instruments were provided, and patients learned to work together as a team in order to perform both in the hospital auditorium and for parades and other events on the grounds.

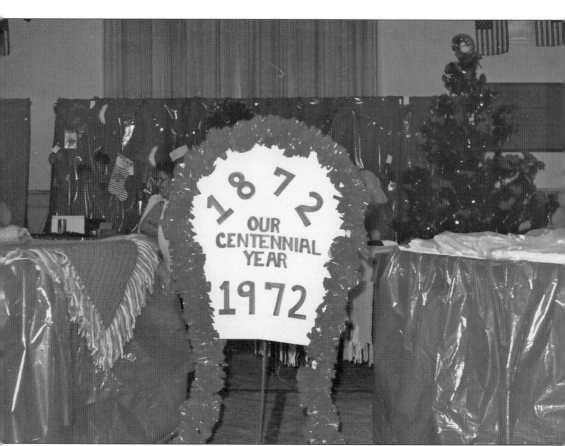

Arts and crafts were made by the patients as form of therapy, but the finished goods served many uses. Some items were used in the hospital center as essential equipment. Other items were given to other public institutions in Essex County. Some items were also sold to the public. Once every year, Overbrook held an event where the public was able to come in and purchase some of these crafts. Crafts were also put up for sale in Newark and other bordering cities. Any money raised during the sales went back to the hospital center. This either funded materials for the recreational therapy department or patient currency. (Courtesy of Robert L. Williams.)

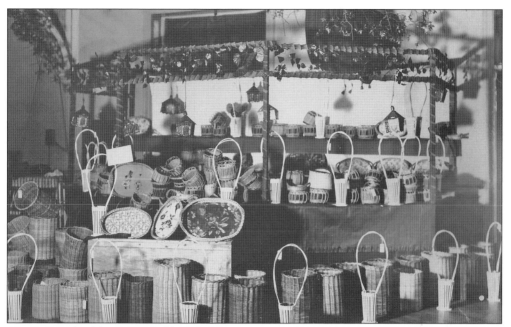

A centennial celebration is held in the Occupational Therapies Building, which was previously directly adjacent to Building 11. Patients and staff offer handmade items for sale ranging from purses to quilts. Proceeds raised from such events would be used to fund various hospital expenses and to purchase necessary supplies.

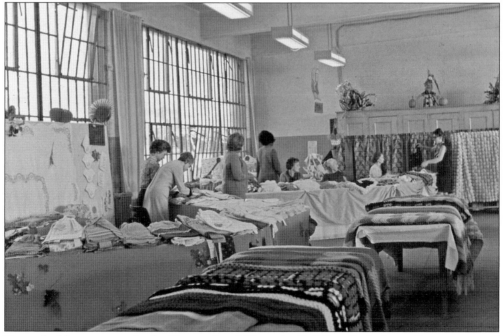

Rows of tables are set up in the Occupational Therapies Building displaying quilts, scarves, and other goods produced by the patients enrolled in the programs. Such events were open to the public and helped strengthen the connection between the patients, faculty, administration, and community.

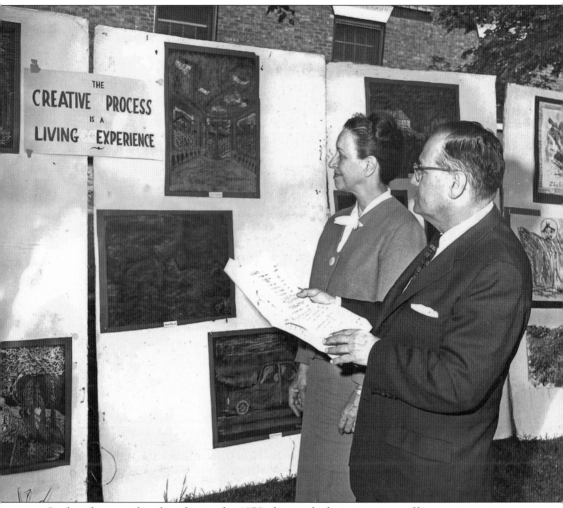

In this photograph, taken during the 1970s, hospital administrative staff compare program notes at an outdoor art exhibition behind the Hill Wards. The exhibit, billed as The Creative Process Is a Living Experience, featured works of art in various formats made by the patients at Overbrook. They were allotted an assortment of arts and crafts supplies and worked with everything from crayons to pastels and various paints. (Courtesy of Newark Public Library.)

Five

TREATMENT AND CONDITIONS

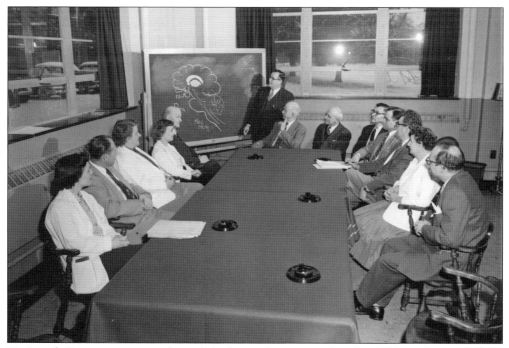

Dr. Joseph Sutton, superintendent of the hospital, is pictured in the 1950s at the head of the table leading an educational meeting with other administrative and doctoral staff. A crude chalk drawing of the anatomy of a brain is presented with emphasis on the pituitary gland and the medulla oblongata. This time period began the introduction of modern psychiatric drugs, including thorazine and other first-generation antipsychotics. Dr. Joseph Sutton passed away on August 5, 1971, at nearby Mountainside Hospital in Montclair. (Courtesy of Newark Public Library.)

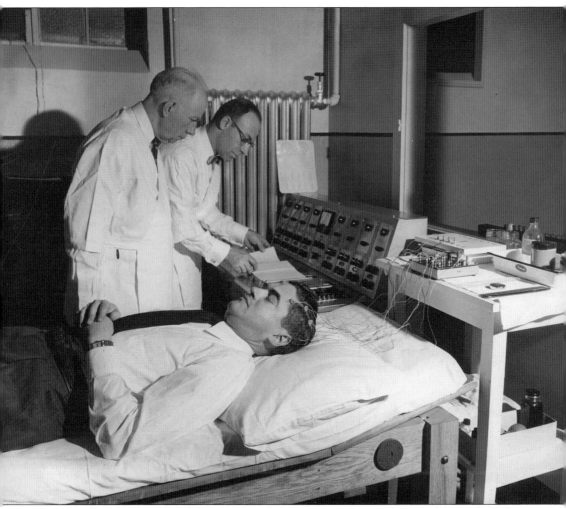

Dr. Joseph Sutton stands at left next to Frank Antonacci as they conduct an electroencephalogram, otherwise known as an EEG. This photograph, taken in the basement of Building 11, was actually set up for demonstrative purposes. Dr. Sutton served as the hospital superintendent and medical director from 1950 until 1957, with Frank Antonacci as the head of the x-ray department. On the table is Charles Mercer, a reporter for the Associated Press. The hospital frequently allowed reporters and photographers to document the advances they were making in medical treatments and patient care. Mercer went on to write an article for the Associated Press that was published in the *Decatur Herald* on April 4, 1954, titled "What Communist Brain-Washing Can Do to a Man." The article references Dr. Sutton's personal experience caring for psychiatric patients. (Courtesy of Newark Public Library.)

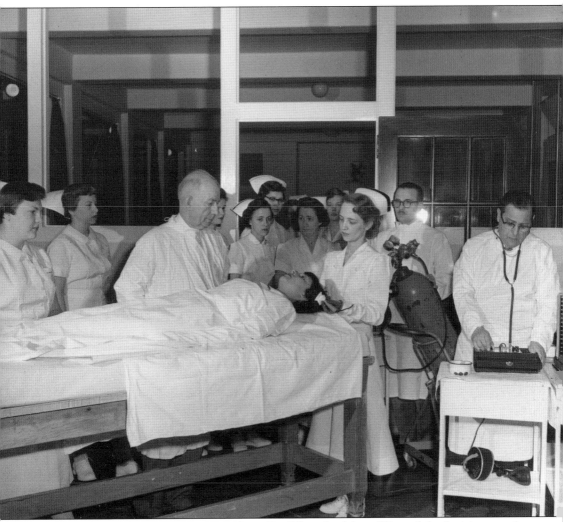

In this photograph are Dr. Henry Davidson, Dr. Wysocki, Mona Kline, Julia Jennings, and Dr. Joseph Sutton demonstrating the use of electroshock therapy on another nurse as students watch. This was another example of posed photographs featured in articles regarding the medical advancements made at Essex County Overbrook Hospital. Charles Mercer, of the Associated Press, would later publish an article using these photographs and firsthand experiences from shadowing Dr. Sutton and Dr. Davidson. One such article can be found in the *Bridgeport Post* from January 30, 1955. The publication goes into great detail regarding the treatments and diagnostics used at the hospital, ranging from lobotomies to the use of psychology to modify behaviors. (Courtesy of Newark Public Library.)

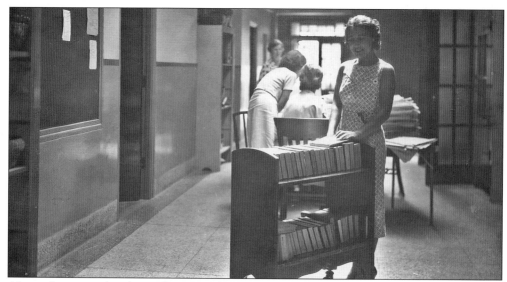

Alongside nurses, female employees in the hospital were employed in both the library and in records rooms. The library was inside Building 7, the service building. It was split into two sections, the patient library and the staff library. The staff library contained medical dictionaries, while the patient library contained the regular categories of publications.

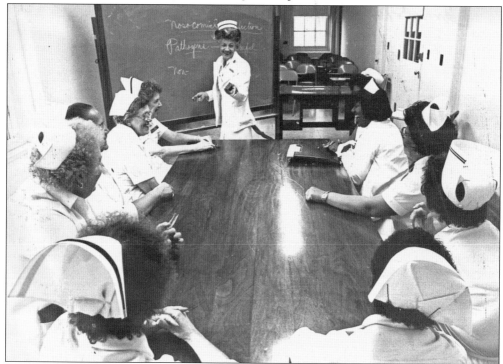

The nurses seen here are attending a meeting on hospital safety in regards to disease and infection control. The lead nurse goes over the definitions of pathogens, such as airborne diseases, as well as nosocomial infections, or diseases originating from the hospital that could spread from patient to patient. During this time period, tuberculosis was being successfully treated and vaccines were becoming readily available, which led to a great reduction in communicable diseases.

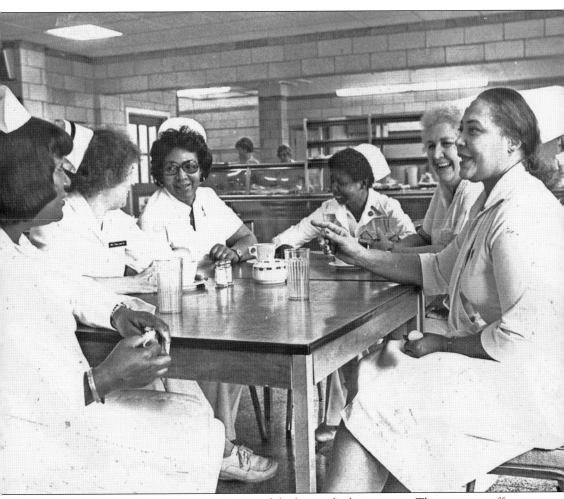

Nurses can be seen enjoying beverages in one of the hospital's dining areas. The support staff at Overbrook Hospital was world renowned for its knowledge and caring attitude. The nursing staff at Overbrook was trained onsite through Overbrook's nursing training program. The nurses stayed onsite in the nurses' cottages on the west side of Fairview Avenue and were there for a period of time as students. Once they graduated from the program, they had the opportunity for full-time employment at Overbrook. The head nurse met with the supervisor of the training program to discuss the candidate's credentials and performance. Overbrook had one of the most highly rated nursing programs in the nation. The program was discontinued in the 1980s, as many individuals were gaining their education through colleges.

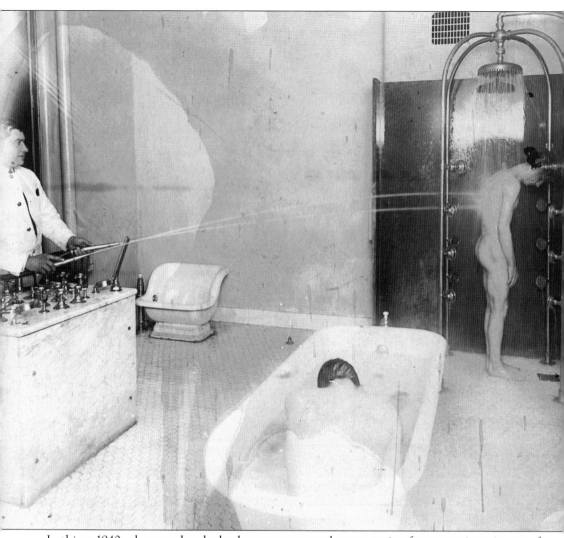

In this c. 1940s photograph, a hydrotherapy nurse can be seen caring for two patients in one of the hospital's many large hydrotherapy treatment facilities, designed as part of a treatment to calm agitated or manic patients before the advent of modern antipsychotics. In a September 1946 article by Harriet J. Smith for the *Des Moines Register*, it is noted that around 50,000 of these treatments and tonic baths were given in 1945. Hydrotherapy consisted of a number of different forms ranging from hot baths with steam to cold baths to shock the patient into compliance, as well as "needle showers," which consisted of many pinpoint showerheads that sprayed water at a high pressure. This was done with the thought that it was a stimulating massage to the internal organs of depressed patients, which might help them feel more energized. The hospital discontinued hydrotherapy in 1957. (Courtesy of Newark Public Library.)

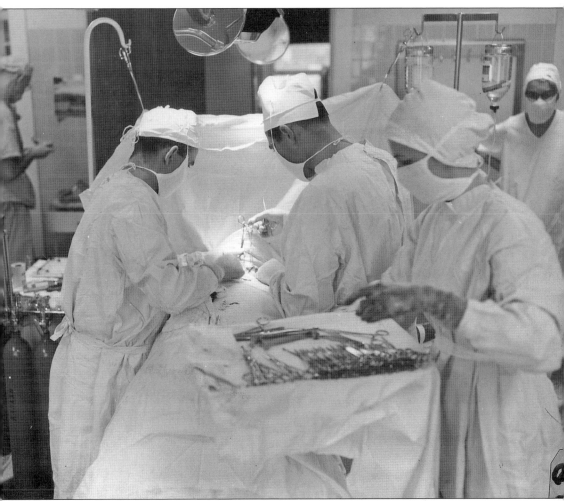

Overbrook Hospital was distinguished for its skilled physicians, who treated not only mental illness but also physical ailments. In this 1954 photograph, a surgeon performs a thyroid operation on a patient. This is just one of over 100 major operations that occurred in the course of a year in the operating room in the Reception Building. The hospital garnered a high reputation for its care of patients and was routinely featured in various publications throughout the United States. This photograph was included in an article titled "What Can Laymen Believe about Mental Health" in the *Courier-Journal* of Louisville, Kentucky. The article goes into detail about the trial and errors of the care associated with psychiatric patients, as well as the gold standard of care they receive under Dr. Joseph Sutton's direction.

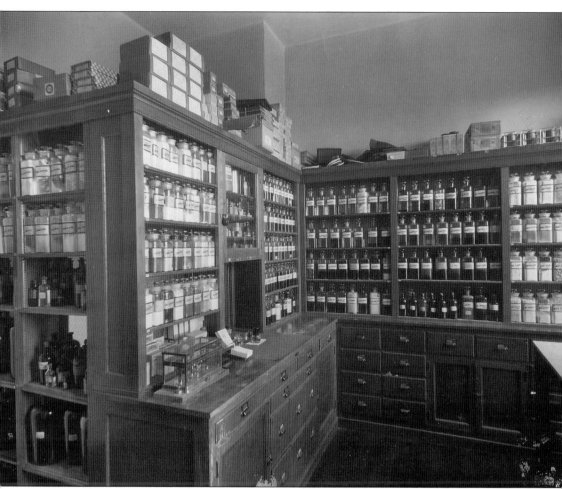

The fully stocked pharmacy in the basement of Building 11 is documented here during the late 1920s. Common household medical supplies still used today can be noted on the far right, ranging from aspirin and boric acid to caffeine, magnesium oxide, gelatin, and potassium bromide, which is still used in veterinary medicine. To the left is a variety of liquids, some stored in amber bottles to protect them from sunlight, including menthol, camphor, and phenol. These products were often applied to the skin to treat sores or as pain relief, since they all work as a topical analgesic. It is also important to note the bottle of chloroform, which was used as an anesthesia inhalant until it was phased out around 1932 in exchange for much safer medications.

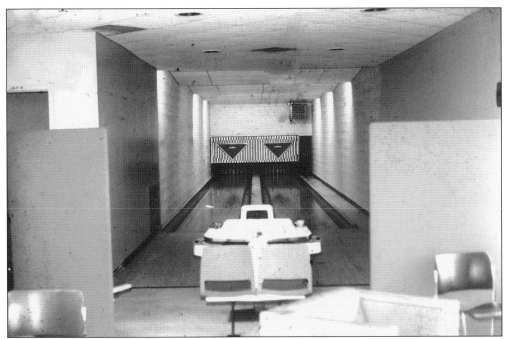

When the new Recreational Therapy Building was constructed in place of the Star Building, it was expected to improve the care of patients through activities. Pictured above is the bowling alley for the hospital. These types of activity treatments became a new style of care at Overbrook once the building was operational. (Courtesy of Justin Gurbisz.)

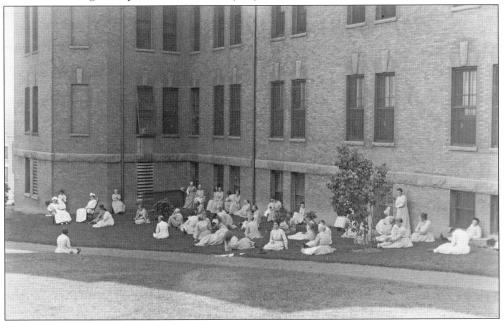

In this photograph from the early 1900s, female patients are seated on the beautifully manicured lawn just outside the Star Building. There were additional gazebo structures set up along the perimeter of the Star Building. This was an attempt to give patients more encouragement to spend time outdoors.

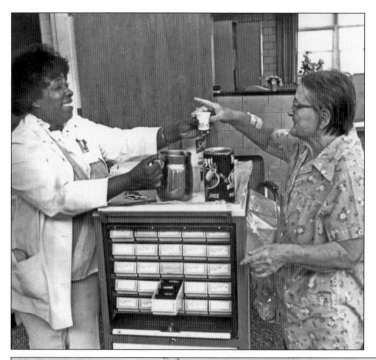

A geriatric patient can be seen receiving her daily medications from a nurse with her choice of apple or orange juice. Her attire is typical of hospital patients, consisting of comfortable clothing that can be easily snapped together in lieu of buttons, which may be more difficult to use for patients with dexterity complications. Psychiatric drugs developed during this time period significantly improved the quality of life for patients at the hospital. (Courtesy of the Newark Public Library.)

Complete Schooling At Hospital

Two exceptional young ladies were among hundreds of teenagers receiving diplomas during the past week at Essex County high school graduation exercises.

The exceptional nature of these two paricular young ladiets, each of them 17-and-a-half years old, was not discernible to the audiences at two of the county's public high schools.

They were quite like all the other girls in their graduating classes. What makes them exceptional is that they are patients (schizophrenics) at Essex County Overbrook Hospital, Cedar Grove. They are members of the hospital's adolescent unit which consists of 20 teenagers — 10 boys and 10 girls, all committed to the hospital for various kinds of mental illness.

The two girls are on extended leave from the hospital and are expected to be discharged in about a year. They still will be patients for that period and will return to the hospital from time to time for group therapy sessions.

One of the girls has applied for admission to a business chool in September and the other is planning to enroll in college, also in the Fall.

The two girls are believed to be the first two such high school graduates in the country.

The hospital's high school is operated by the Cedar Grove board of education. Cedar Grove pays the salaries of the teachers and in turn compensated with funds from the school districts in which the teen-age patients normally reside. All the equipment and supplies for the "school within a hospital" also are supplied by Cedar Grove.

The adolescent unit was started on April 8, 1963 and the school was established several months later. For the past school year it has been accredited by the state board of education.

The adolescent unit is the only one in the state connected with a public mental hospital. It is also one of the first of its kind in the United States. There still are only half a dozen such units in the country.

The "school within a hospital" is the first in the country to become an integral unit of a public school system. There are seven public mental hospitals in New Jersey, two county and five state hospitals, and about 200 public

This publication, featured in the July 1, 1965, *Verona–Cedar Grove Times*, describes the drastic improvement of two particular adolescent patients at Overbrook Hospital. In order to serve the community better, a unit was created in 1963 to care for children and teenagers. Essex County was a pioneer in this regard, as it was one of the first to be conceived in the United States and the only one in New Jersey.

MURDER INDICTMENT FOUND AGAINST NOEL

Essex Grand Jury Also Charges Him With Kidnapping Mary Daly.

HAD NO AID, POLICE THINK

Dr. Thompson Denies Blame for Escape—Inquiries to Fix Responsibility Begin.

Harrison Noel, escaped lunatic and confessed slayer of six-year-old Mary Daly and Raymond Pierce, was indicted by the Essex County Grand Jury yesterday for the murder of Pierce and for the kidnapping of the child. No indictment for the murder of the child was found, because that crime was committed in Passaic County.

An investigation to discover whether Noel had an accomplice in his series of crimes established the fact that occasionally over two years Noel had called himself by the name of Wallace Payne, which is also the name of a mentally defective criminal who escaped a year ago from a New York State institution at Napanoch, Ulster County.

Further investigations were started yesterday to discover whether Noel's father or the authorities of the Overbrook institution created the opportunity for the crime by conniving at the continued freedom of the escaped youth.

Accomplice Theory Questioned.

The theory that Noel had an accomplice named Wallace Payne received a setback yesterday when two employes of the postoffice at Little Falls identified photographs of Noel as the man who had received mail there under the name of Wallace Payne. Noel called himself Wallace Payne when he claimed the package containing the pistol which was mailed to Wallace Payne. According to Postmaster Morehouse and his clerk, Julia Dixon, Noel had appeared there at other times during the past two years calling himself Wallace Payne.

Whether Noel knew the lunatic Payne, or whether Noel's adoption of that name was merely a coincidence, puzzled the investigators yesterday. Several things suggested that Noel might have had an accomplice. Payne's whereabouts are now unknown. Payne was arrested on two different occasions for attacks on young girls. He was rated as possessing 70 per cent. of the normal mental capacity, according to Dr. Walter N. Thayer, Superintendent of the Institution for Defective Delinquents at Napanoch, from which Payne escaped a year ago.

"I don't know that Noel ever knew Payne," said Dr. Thayer. "It's possible that they met. Payne might have been capable of cooperating with Noel in these crimes, and Noel's use of Payne's name is a singular coincidence, if they were not acquainted. Payne was not, properly speaking, insane, but was deficient."

Dr. Thayer said that his institution and other institutions had no special machinery to set in motion to trace fugitives.

"We have to send out descriptions and rely on the police," he said. "There is no special agency at our service for recapturing runaways."

James Carpenter of Jersey City, lawyer for Dix W. Noel, father of Harrison Noel, said yesterday that he had no information that Noel was ever acquainted with any Wallace Payne. H. C. Barber, spokesman for the Noel family, said last night that it was known that young Noel was at one time in the neighborhood of the Napanoch institution, but that the family had not learned whether he made the acquaintance of Payne.

Might Have Had Accomplice.

Captain James Mason of the Essex County Prosecutor's detective staff and Chief of Police Reilly of Montclair were skeptical of the theory that Noel had an accomplice, because of the fact that when he started confessing Noel seemingly confessed in full. None of his statements has been found to be false. He denied that he had any assistance of any kind.

They admitted, however, that there were two circumstances which pointed

Continued on Page Three.

MURDER INDICTMENT FOUND AGAINST NOEL

Continued from Page 1, Column 4.

in the other direction. The first was that Mrs. William J. Bogan of Cedar Grove, who took the car's number when she became suspicious on seeing it stopped for a long time on a lonely road, was sure that she saw two men—one being Noel and the other a man crouched down in the rear seat so that she could see little of him. As Mrs. Bogan's powers of observation led directly to the arrest of Noel, her positiveness that she saw an accomplice had carried a good deal of weight. Mrs. Bogan's statement is supported to some extent by the circumstances under which the body of Pierce was found. The negro weighed more than 200 pounds. Noel is less than 150 and looks weak. Yet the body of the negro was removed 200 feet from the road. From indications, it was carried clear of the ground. There was no sign of a path through the grass caused by dragging the body.

It was reported that a Wallace Payne had once lived at Little Falls. This caused Chief of Police Dougherty of that place to go through the tax records and other records, but he found no trace of such a person.

The Essex County Board of Freeholders will meet at Newark this morning to find out who was responsible for the fact that an admittedly insane man, who had already made three murderous attempts, was allowed to go free to commit two more.

Doctor Denies Blame.

Dr. John M. Thompson, senior surgeon of the Overbrook Hospital, from which young Noel escaped, made an emphatic denial yesterday of the statement that he had failed to demand the return of the fugitive and had encouraged the father to keep the boy at home. He asserted that the blame for continuing the boy at large rested solely on the father.

"I knew that Harrison Noel could never recover," he said, "but his father is a very domineering man who came to me, not for advice or suggestions—he would not entertain them—but to tell me how well his son was getting along. At certain intervals the boy knew right from wrong, but at other times he lost control of himself completely.

"When I realized Harrison Noel's father did not intend to bring the boy back, I told him it was a duty he owed to the State, to society, to the hospital, to me, and to himself to return him. After that conversation, he promised to bring him back at two o'clock the next afternoon. I heard from him the next afternoon, but by telephone, and he told me that Harrison had put in such a good night he did not think he would bring him back to the hospital.

"He evidently decided to play the part of physician as well as father. I couldn't get hold of him after that. Harrison Noel should have been brought back under the wing of this institution. Dix W. Noel asked me nothing. He knew more about the boy's case than Overbrook knew. I believe that if the boy had remained at Bellevue Hospital, they would have turned him over to us, but the father evidently put up one of his grand arguments and effected the boy's release.

"In all the time Harrison Noel was under my observation he never displayed any feeling. He was what is classed as a 'shut-in' boy. He would listen, but he would give no reply. He would always do opposite to what he was told. But I got along with him very nicely, probably because I am a Harvard man and he once attended Harvard.

"I never said the boy would recover, because I knew he could never recover. Dix W. Noel is a man of fixed opinions and a domineering nature. I was honest in my observations and I told him the boy should be sent back to us. But the father controlled him. We realized the significance of Harrison Noel's escape and we believed he should be brought back.

"It is a downright shame for Noel to treat me as he has. If he had kept his promise and returned the boy there would have been no crime. I do not want to antagonize Noel, but the records of the hospital show what happened. These records have been turned over to the Freeholders. Noel was steering the boat—he didn't give me a chance.

"That boy was never in fit shape to take up outside employment, and I never said he was."

Dr. Guy Payne, Superintendent of the Hospital at Overbrook, said yesterday that he knew nothing of any authorization for the father to keep the boy instead of returning him to the institution.

"I don't know of Mr. Noel having any communication with the hospital authorities after the escape of his son," he said.

The charge that New Jersey institutions have generally been lax in releasing lunatics was followed yesterday by the charge on responsible authority that New York State was freeing men of the Noel type because there was no room for them in New York State institutions. This assertion came from Dr. Marcus B. Heyman, Superintendent of Manhattan State Hospital at Ward's Island.

"We are forced," he said, "to free such men as these two (Harrison Noel and Stanley Krynovoak, who killed a man Tuesday on Staten Island) on parole to make room for patients whose mental condition we consider even more dangerous.

"Crimes committed by insane persons will go on unabated until the citizens of New York State pass the $100,000,000 bond issue, which comes up for their vote in the November election. A part of this money will be used for the construction of additional buildings, so that we can cut down the number of paroled patients and at the same time admit the thousands of known insane who are walking the streets of the cities and villages of the State of New York.

"What is true of conditions at the Manhattan State Hospital is true also of conditions in the other thirteen State institutions for the care of the insane."

Vigorous Reform Urged.

Vigorous handling of the problem of the so-called "harmless lunatics," responsible for so many atrocious crimes, was urged yesterday by Commissioner of Institutions Burdette G. Lewis of New Jersey, formerly Commissioner of Correction in this city. He urged that the reform should begin with the routine neurological examination of children in public schools, like the present routine dental and optical examinations. He asserted that most murderers of the young gunman type presented symptoms of mental disease at school age, and that most of them could be treated and cured if taken in time.

Commissioner Lewis said that the New Jersey institutions for the insane were, on the whole, severe in their precautions against escape and against the premature release of inmates in doubtful cases.

"The Overbrook institution has in recent months shown a great improvement in its management," he said, "and I would be sorry to find that it has been at fault in this case, if that is so.

"The menace of the unrecognized lunatic and of doubtful cases is one of the most serious ones which society has to deal with. I believe that present methods are unsatisfactory in all parts of the country, and that what is needed is an awakening on the part of the people to the necessity for dealing with this question in a serious and thorough manner, beginning with the children in the schools. Most of our murderers and other criminals showed signs in childhood of mental troubles which can be detected by specialists and treated.

"I believe the State should step in and assert its right to diagnose and treat such cases in spite of the opposition which is aroused at every step in that direction. The cry is that personal liberty is being violated and that the home is being invaded every time any effort is made to secure legislation which would enable the State to deal with a lunatic who has not demonstrated his lunacy by some crime or public exhibition of his unbalanced condition. At present public sentiment is against scientific handling of this problem. This is shown whenever actions are brought to obtain freedom for lunatics. If the man looks all right and shows some intelligence the jury usually voted to free him regardless of the fact that he may have a taint which is likely to break out again in a short time."

Noel Still Apathetic.

Noel has not talked with attendants or given any signs of remorse or other reaction, it was said at the Essex County Jail, where he is confined in a "double-cage" cell. His lawyer was forbidden to visit him today. Permission was given to the family to bring clothes to him on Friday, the visiting day. The father may see the boy on that day if he desires.

"I have advised him not to," said Mr. Carpenter, the father's lawyer. "I think it would be better for both of them if they do not see each other then."

The father will not make any attempt to keep his son out of an institution for the insane, according to the lawyer.

"Mr. Noel has no thought of having his son released," he said. "He feels that the boy is insane and a dangerous person to have loose."

The indictments returned against Harrison Noel yesterday will probably be presented in the court of Oyer and Terminer before Judge Edwin C. Caffrey on Saturday, Acting Prosecutor J. Victor D'Aloia said.

The charge of murdering the child and of assaulting John Sandin, who pursued the kidnaping car and was shot in the head, rest with Passaic County, since both crimes were committed in that county. These charges will in all probability be brought before the Passaic County Grand Jury in Paterson on Sept. 22.

The acting prosecutor said last night that young Noel probably will plead to two indictments next Wednesday. New Jersey law requires that a trial be held within two weeks after the prisoner has pleaded.

Negroes in Montclair have started a movement to collect funds for the destitute family of Raymond Pierce, the murdered taxi driver. In addition to the widow, there are four small children. Director of Public Safety Robinson of Montclair said that the town might take care of the family. Captain James Mason of the Essex County Prosecutor's office had another suggestion.

"If all the people who are trying to claim the $3,250 reward for the slayer's capture would agree to turn it over to the Pierce family," the captain said, "I would gladly resign all claim to it."

Mrs. Bogan, wife of the Chief of Police of Cedar Grove, who gave police the number of the Noel automobile, which she saw in Van Geisen's gap on the morning of the kidnapping, has filed claim to the reward with the Montclair Town Commission.

SLAYER PLEADS NOT GUILTY.

Adds That if He Hadn't Shot Man He Would Have Gone Crazy.

Stephen Krynovoak, 24 years old, of 116 Cedar Street, Stapleton, S. I., who was paroled from the Manhattan Insane Asylum on Aug. 29 and shot Adam Lukaski, a delicatessen dealer, of 143 Tompkins Street, Stapleton, Tuesday, alleging that the man had struck his mother seven years ago, showed no emotion yesterday when he pleaded not guilty to the charge of murder before Magistrate Bridges in the New Brighton Police Court.

"If I had not killed him," said Krynovoak gravely, "I would have gone crazy."

He was held without bail for examination next Wednesday. Charles Bergoff, his attorney, said he may ask County Judge Tiernan to appoint a sanity commission for Krynovoak.

In September 1925, a double homicide rattled Cedar Grove and nearby communities. Harrison W. Noel, 20 years old at the time, hailed a cab in the vicinity of the Montclair railroad station, commonly known now as Lackawanna Terminal. He then shot cab driver Raymond Pierce in the back of the head with a small pistol he had purchased only days earlier. Two days later, Pierce's body was found in Cedar Grove near the Peckman River, not far from the hospital center. After killing and disposing of Pierce, Noel went on to kidnap six-year-old Mary Daly in front of her Montclair home for a $4,000 ransom. However, he inexplicably changed his mind and shot Daly in the head, dumping her body in Little Falls. Noel had previously been a patient at Overbrook but escaped and was never recommitted. The ensuing controversy surrounding Noel's family, as well as statements from Dr. John M. Thompson, senior surgeon for the hospital, were heavily documented in the *New York Times*.

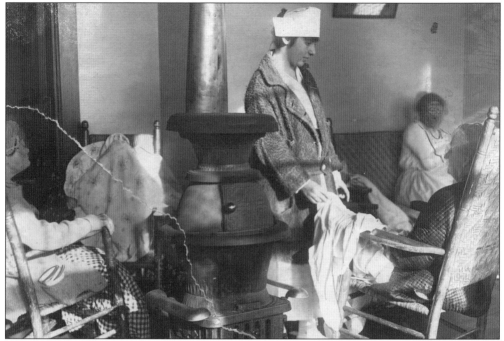

Dated December 17, 1917, this photograph depicts a nurse caring for her charges in one of the hospital's many dayrooms. During this time period, the main boilers had a malfunction and stopped working. Temperatures were only a few degrees above freezing, and Dr. Guy Payne urged family members to pick up their loved ones. During this time, 24 deaths related to the cold occurred in 20 days. (Courtesy of Newark Public Library.)

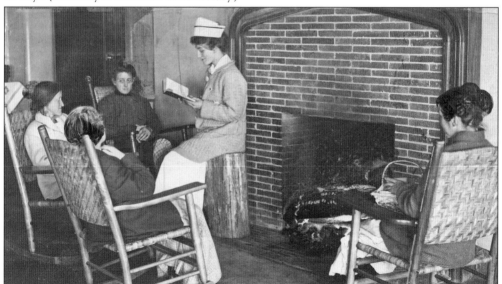

This view of another dayroom, taken on December 27, 1917, shows a group of female patients swathed in coats and sweaters sitting before an open fireplace. The brick fireplaces were a prominent feature in the hospital's architecture and were highlighted in photographs even during its period of abandonment. A nurse can be seen sitting in the midst of the group reading a story during this relaxing moment. (Courtesy of the Newark Public Library.)

Mrs. Ward takes notes from a geriatric patient as a colleague looks on. Mrs. Ward was the head nurse for the Wright Pavilion and also did some work at the Essex County Isolation Hospital in Belleville. The Isolation Hospital was later shifted towards geriatric care as part of the Essex County Hospital System. (Courtesy of the Newark Public Library.)

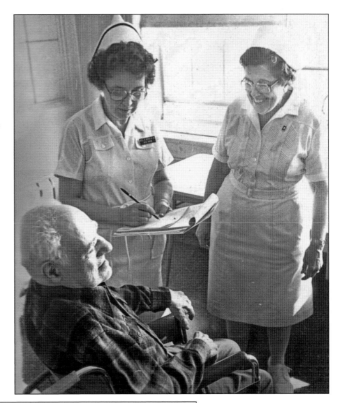

Result at Overbrook

Care of Patients Improved

The quality of patient care has improved in the past four months in a number of wards at Overbrook Hospital as a result of participation in a Health Occupational Training (HOT) program.

This appraisal was made by hospital officials and representatives of the Hospital Research and Educational Trust of New Jersey, a co-sponsor of the program with the United States Department of Labor's Bureau of Apprenticeship and Training.

The success of the first phase of the program, which began Sept. 18 and provided 840 hours of classroom and clinical instruction for 76 attendants, has led to a new contract between HOT and Overbrook. It provides for a full year of on-the-job training of 140 semi-skilled and unskilled ward attendants.

On-Job Training

Basic psychiatric and general skills, to enable attendants to assist doctors and nurses in providing better patient care, will be emphasized, according to Dr. Henry A. Davidson, superintendent and medical director.

Mrs. Catherine B. Finnerty and Mrs. Dolores Van Dessel, registered nurses and instructors, pointed out that only 15 per cent of the program has been classroom teaching. Follow-up clinical instruction in wards constituted the other 85 per cent.

Also involved in the program are the New Jersey Employment Service and Total Employment and Manpower, Inc., (TEAM), Newark's "Concentrated Employment Program."

Overbrook was one of the first two mental hospitals in the state to participate in HOT, the other being Trenton State Hospital. Overbrook is the largest county-operated mental institute in the nation and one of only two county-operated psychiatric institutions in the country with full national accreditation.

The program is supported by federal funds provided by the Manpower Development and Training Act, which was designed to give job skills to the unemployed and technologically displaced. The instructors' salaries and various types of visual aids are provided by the program.

This newspaper clipping, dated January 21, 1968, details the many advancements taking place at the hospital. Essex County Overbrook Hospital was the largest county-operated mental institution in the nation at this time and one of only two with full accreditation. After the retirement of Dr. Joseph Sutton, Dr. Henry Davidson, who previously worked alongside Dr. Sutton for many years, stepped up to the position of superintendent and medical director. (Courtesy of Newark Public Library.)

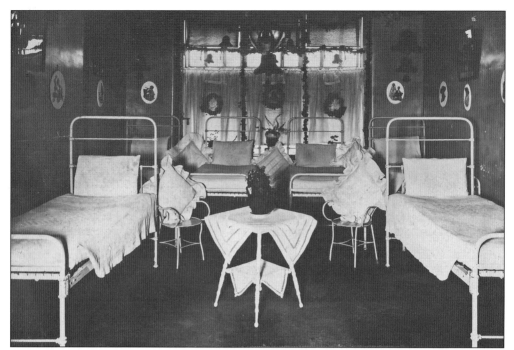

The large patient room seen in this early-20th-century photograph has been decorated for the holiday season. Nonviolent and nondisruptive patients were frequently housed together in rooms consisting of up to a dozen or so beds. These wards were occupied by only one gender, with men and women being housed in completely separate buildings. (Courtesy of Robert L. Williams.)

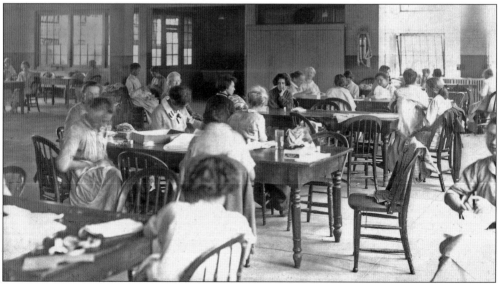

The occupational therapies offered by Overbrook were often based upon gender. In this photograph, women can be seen participating in a sewing class. The various blankets, clothing, handbags, and costumes produced by the occupational therapies patients were used in the hospital and sold to members of the community. These classes helped people learn important life skills in the hopes that once they were well enough to be released, they could be gainfully employed right away. (Courtesy of Robert L. Williams.)

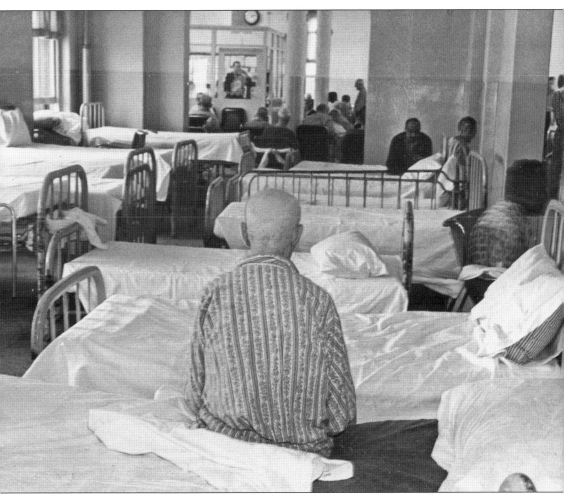

During the 1960s and early 1970s, patient overcrowding became a problem at the hospital center. A male patient of the Star Building looks at the dozens of beds that occupy his ward. The Star Building held the hospital's most violent and dangerous patients in the later years of the building's life. The Star Building had been plagued with criticism for many years, dating back to a September 15, 1934, article in the *New York Times* describing it as a "firetrap." Henry C. Miller, foreman of a grand jury convened to analyze complaints of this particular building, was quoted as saying "as soon as finances allow . . . the building ought to be rebuilt." The Star Building was eventually demolished in 1978, just four years after this photograph was published. (Courtesy of Newark Public Library.)

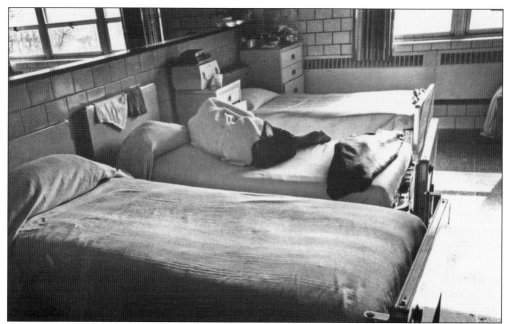

A depressed patient lies down on a modern hospital bed on the second floor of the Reception Building. Patients who did not pose a threat to themselves or others were regularly allowed to freely dress themselves in their own clothing and keep personal possessions at their bedside. Overbrook was the only facility in Essex County that was equipped for long-term-stay care. (Courtesy of Newark Public Library.)

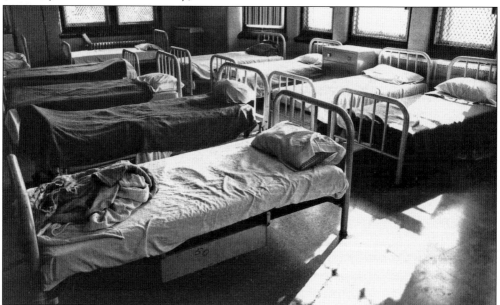

Open dormitories housing multiple occupants in the Hill Buildings became the norm during the 1970s until the eventual closure of some wards. Patients were allowed access to their own wardrobes and drawers to house some of their personal belongings as well as hospital-issued clothing. The striped window shades visible here remained in place for many years to come and can be seen in modern photographs of the hospital's abandonment. (Courtesy of Newark Public Library.)

Six

CLOSURE AND
ABANDONMENT

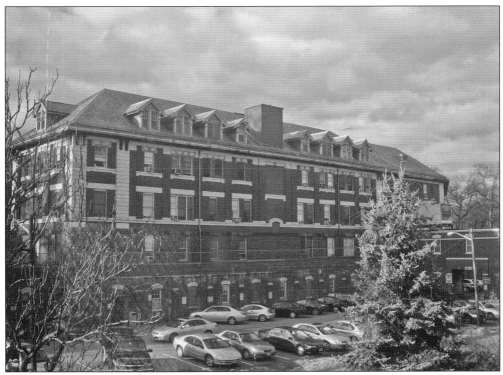

By 2006, a new state-of-the-art hospital center had been constructed directly behind Overbrook on Grove Avenue. The remaining Overbrook patients were transferred to the new hospital in February 2007, marking the closure of this historic facility. Employees were also moved over to the new facility, and Overbrook was sealed up and left to rot. Above is one of the last times the Administration Building saw a parking lot filled with cars, shortly before its closure in the winter of 2007. (Photograph by Rob Berner.)

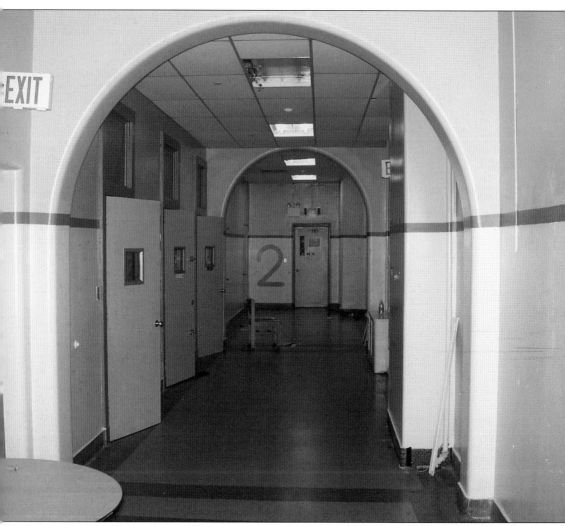

Immediately after closure, the hospital remained in great shape and had the potential for reuse. This corridor is located in Hill Building 3 and connects to Hill Building 2 at the end of the hallway. This section was occupied by employees rather than patients. The number on the wall indicates that the passageway to the left leads to Building 2. The modernization of the hospital is obvious in this photograph. The walls were painted in tranquil colors such as turquoise. It was thought that these colors would help ease the mind. Unfortunately, this hallway fell victim to vandalism years after the hospital's closure. (Photograph by Rob Berner.)

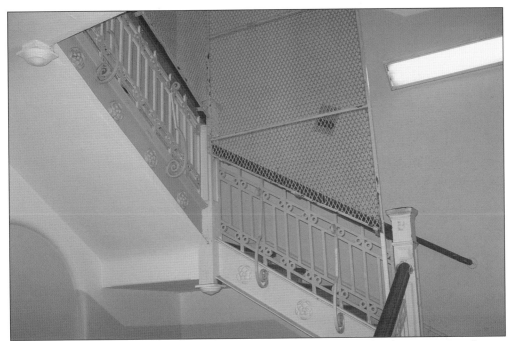

Hill Building 3, the Rehabilitation Wards, had a centralized staircase that became a main feature in photographs of the hospital center after its abandonment. The staircase connected all three floors of the building and featured a cage that ran up the entire length of the staircase. The cage was to prevent patients from jumping down the staircase as a means of suicide. Above is a photograph of the staircase in 2007. (Photograph by Rob Berner.)

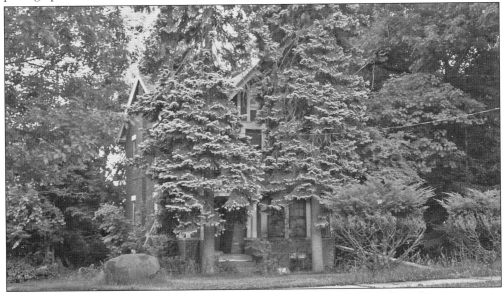

The gardener's home was located along Fairview Avenue, hidden behind two large pine trees. This small two-story home with attic and basement is where the keeper of the greenhouse would reside. The two pine trees can still be seen today when driving down Fairview Avenue. The home was abandoned with the greenhouse, and both were demolished in 2010. (Photograph by Rob Berner.)

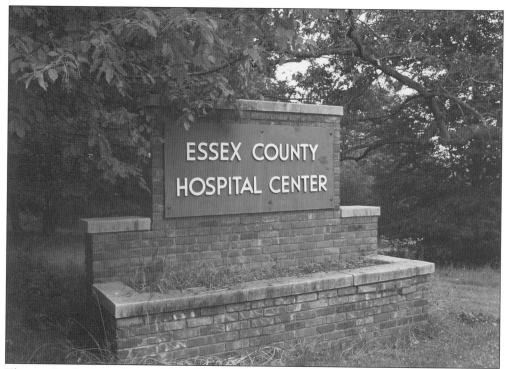

The sign for the Essex County Hospital Center is pictured in 2007. There was an identical sign at each end of Fairview Avenue where the property began and ended. The plaques fell victim to theft in the early years of the hospital's abandonment. The brick structures holding the signs remained standing until the current developer removed them in 2016. (Photograph by Daniel Runyan.)

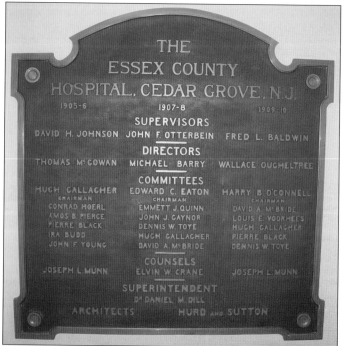

This large steel plaque was located inside the Administration Building. The plaque can be seen in the 1914 photograph in chapter 2. The plaque covered the years 1905 to 1910 and showcased the names of key personnel during this time. It is also important to note the architects behind the hospital center, Hurd and Sutton. This photograph was taken in 2007; the plaque was stolen from the hospital center shortly thereafter. (Photograph by Rob Berner.)

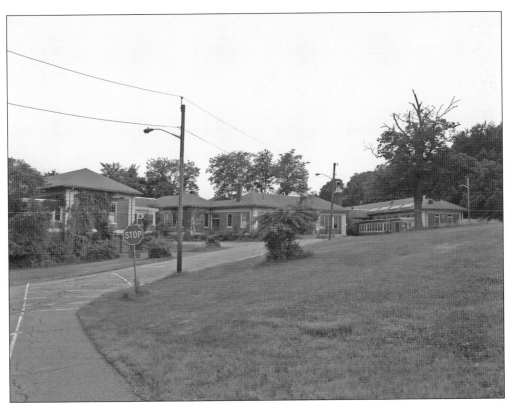

The Freeman Pavilion sits in a state of abandonment in 2007. By the time this building was closed, its main purpose was to house outpatient facilities and business enterprises. At its closure, records from all over the county were being stored behind its walls. This building was cleaned out and demolished shortly after the hospital center closed. (Photograph by Daniel Runyan.)

After the close of Overbrook in 2007, the copper and cupolas were removed from the Hill Buildings. This photograph shows a cupola being removed in 2008. The removal of these historic elements left large holes in the roofs of the buildings. This eventually led to severe water and environmental damage from exposure to the elements, and the condition of the buildings rapidly deteriorated. (Photograph by Rob Berner.)

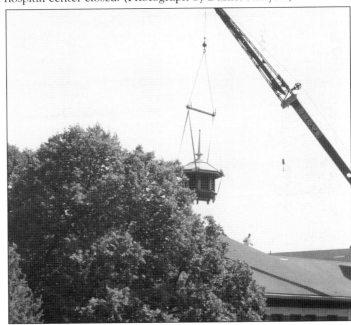

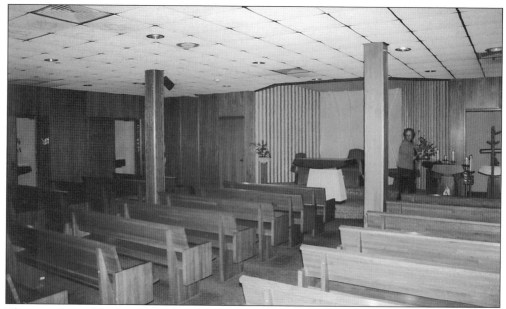

This rare view of the hospital's chapel was taken immediately after closure in 2007. The chapel was used mostly as a synagogue, as a large number of patients at the hospital were Jewish. The chapel was located in Building 7, the service building. The service building was a small structure added on to the connecting breezeway between Hill Building 3 and the Administration Building. (Photograph by Robert L. Williams.)

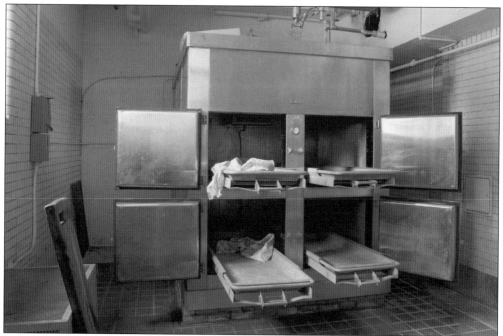

The hospital's four-chamber body freezer sat in the basement of Building 11, the Reception Wards. The morgue was featured in many photographs after the hospital closed. This photograph was taken in 2007 by John Walker of Abandoned New York. John was able to capture the morgue before it fell victim to severe vandalism in later years. (Photograph by John Walker of AbandonedNY.com.)

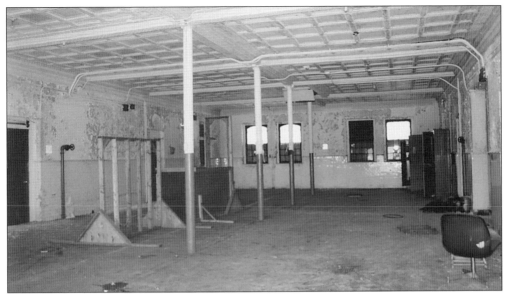

This photograph gives an interior view of the 1915 firehouse building on the west side of Fairview Avenue. The building featured a pole used by firemen to slide down into the garage where the fire engines were parked. There was initially talk of preserving this building, as it was structurally stable and had a cornerstone showcasing the date of 1915. The building was the first to be demolished in 2016. (Photograph by Robert L. Williams.)

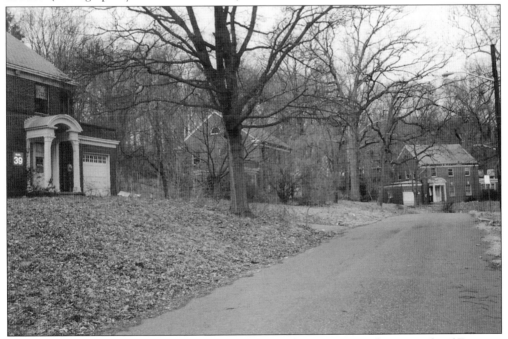

Doctor's Row was on the northern end of the hospital's property on the west side of Fairview Avenue. This stretch of road featured six doctors' homes and a garage used for storage. These buildings were abandoned in the 1980s, when it became impractical for hospital staff to live on campus. All of the homes were demolished by 2010, and this area became part of the Hilltop Reservation and eventually the Cedar Grove Park. (Photograph by Robert L. Williams.)

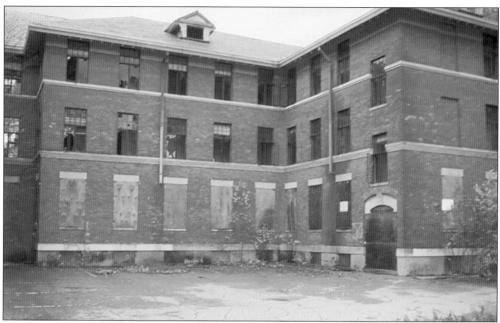

The female employees' home was already in bad condition by the time the hospital closed, as seen in this 2006 photograph. This building was iconic, in that it had a tunnel that ran underground to the main hospital campus. The tunnel crossed under busy Fairview Avenue. When the west side of the campus was demolished, the tunnel was bricked off. (Photograph by Patrick Hayes.)

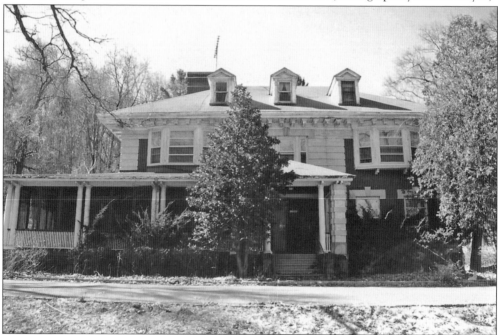

The superintendent's mansion is seen after its abandonment in 2007. This building was home to many stunning pieces of architecture, from the layout of the building to the pieces of furniture inside the home. Many items were salvaged by historian Robert L. Williams before the building's demolition in 2009. (Photograph by Robert L. Williams.)

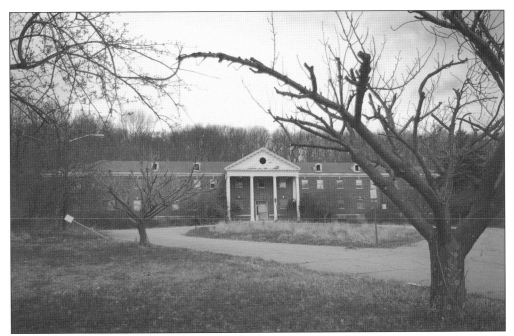

The PEER building was the last of the buildings on the west side of Fairview Avenue to stand. This part of the Overbrook property became part of the Hilltop Reservation, which is the grounds of the former Essex Mountain Sanatorium. In 2017, this entire portion of the property became Cedar Grove Park. (Photograph by Antiquity Echoes.)

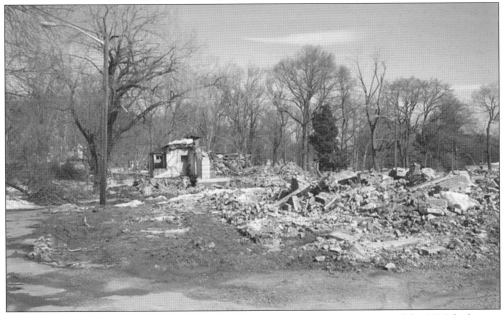

All of the buildings on the west side of Fairview Avenue, with the exception of the 1915 firehouse, were demolished by the end of 2011. The land was left undeveloped until the summer of 2016, when Essex County began to clear the land for the new Cedar Grove Park. The only existing structures that remain in the park are two wells, marked with blue numbered signs, that were used by the hospital. (Photograph by Patrick Hayes.)

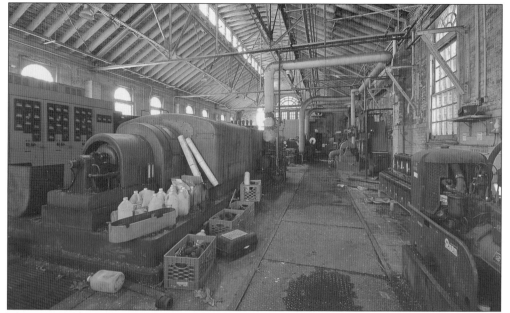

The generating room was one of the only sections of building architecture of the hospital center that remained original to its inception in the early 1900s. The generators and turbines that created steam and heat for the hospital center sat in disuse for years until the building began to be cleaned out for demolition. (Photograph by Justin Gurbisz.)

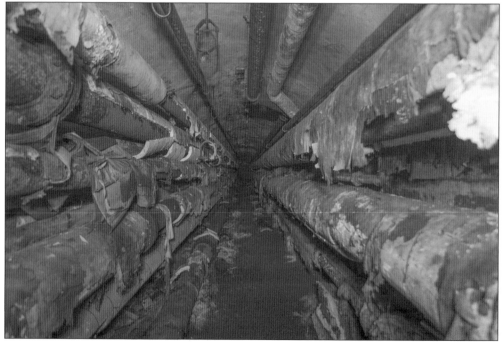

The tunnel system leading out from the powerhouse was a maze of underground passageways that ran for miles. The tunnels provided a means for pipes to run steam and electricity from the powerhouse to the other buildings on campus. After abandonment, the tunnels became a hazard with flooding and falling asbestos pipe coverings. (Photograph by Kevin Kowalick.)

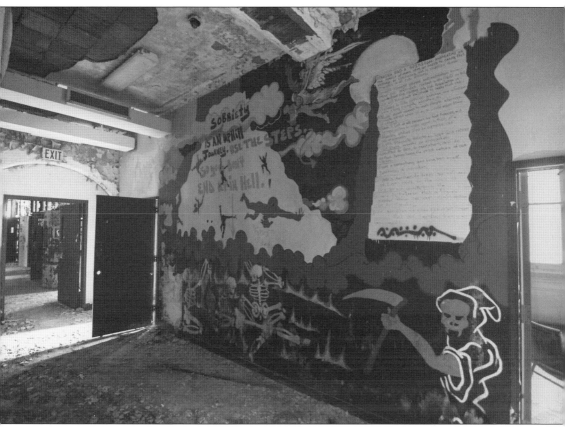

The MICA Wards were located in a structure attached to Hill Building 5. This part of the hospital had murals on the walls promoting sobriety and a positive lifestyle. This mural became iconic after the hospital's closure. It reads, "Sobriety is an uphill journey. Use the steps, so you don't end up in hell." To the right of the text is a small write up about how the patients used certain steps to better their life and end destructive behavior and habits. The imagery shows angels above the clouds followed by individuals falling downwards through the clouds. At the bottom of the image is the patients' visualization of hell with fire, skeletons, and the grim reaper. This mural was painted by the patients and offered a glimpse into what they pictured in their minds. (Photograph by Kevin Kowalick.)

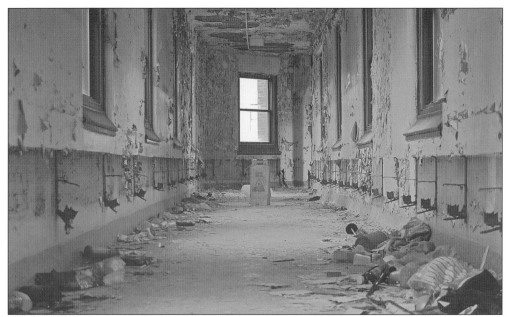

A 2012 view shows the fireproof connector hallways that connected the Hill Buildings. This particular hallway connected Hill Building 3 to Hill Building 4. Below the hallways was an underground passageway that also connected the buildings' basements. The hallway portrayed in this photograph has the original architecture from construction. (Photograph by Justin Gurbisz.)

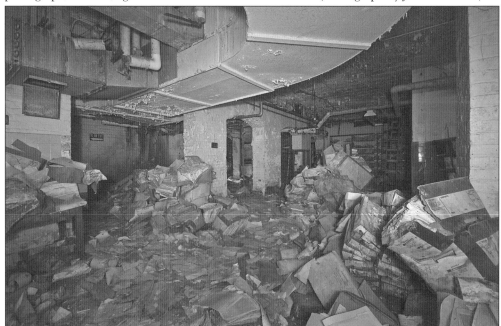

This is one of three records rooms in the basement of Hill Building 3. These records rooms contained documents including patient records, discharges, death files, hospital expenditures, and anything else related to the hospital's operations. Some records from the Essex Mountain Sanatorium and the Essex County Penitentiary were kept at Overbrook as well. Seen here are boxes of records rotting inside the abandoned hospital center. (Photograph by Justin Gurbisz.)

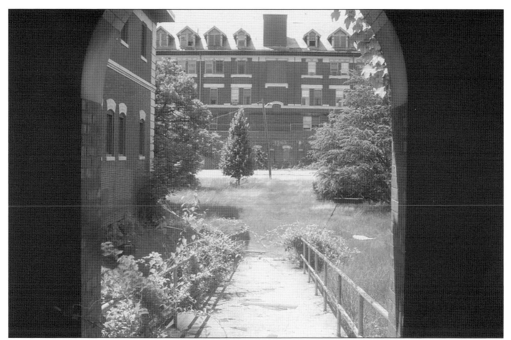

The back of the Administration Building loomed on a higher level of ground above the Hill Buildings. The area between the back of the Administration Building and the back of the Hill Buildings was commonly referred to as the courtyard. Large grassy areas with picnic tables and benches were common in the courtyard to allow patients and staff more space to spend time outdoors. (Photograph by Patrick Hayes.)

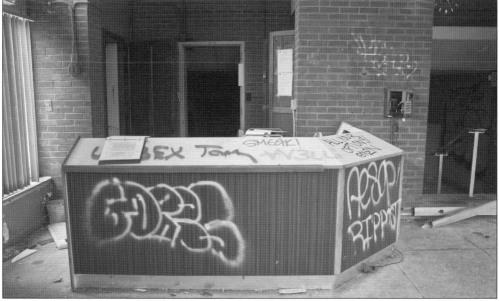

The main entrance to the Administration Building was heavily vandalized after the hospital's closure. The front desk can be seen in this photograph. Here, a security officer would sit and check in everyone who came into the hospital. This area was added in the 1960s. A stairwell to the original part of the building can be seen at right. (Photograph by Kathryn Cataldo.)

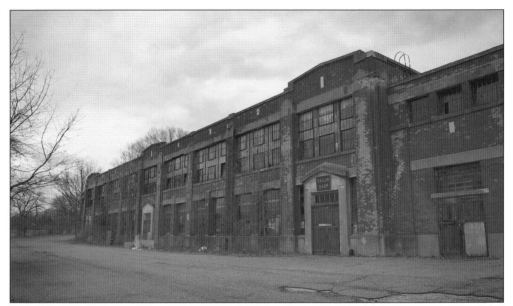

The Occupational Therapies Building is pictured in 2009. This building was never remodeled and held all the original architecture from its construction in the early 1900s. The building was next to Building 11. In 2010, this was one of the few buildings that had been demolished on the east side of Fairview Avenue. Molded sculptures from the patients were dumped in the woods behind the powerhouse. (Photograph by Antiquity Echoes.)

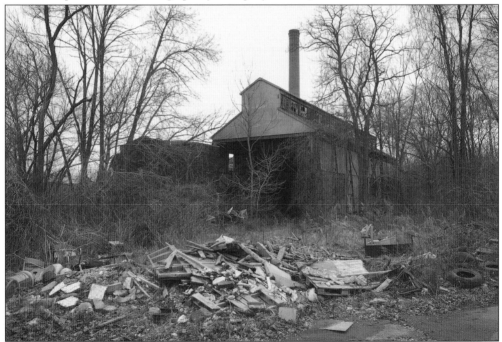

The original coal receiving tipple of the powerhouse stood for many years after closure. The section of the building was decommissioned after the removal of the railroad in the late 1970s. It sat as seen in this 2009 photograph until it collapsed in 2015 due to heavy snowfall. (Photograph by Antiquity Echoes.)

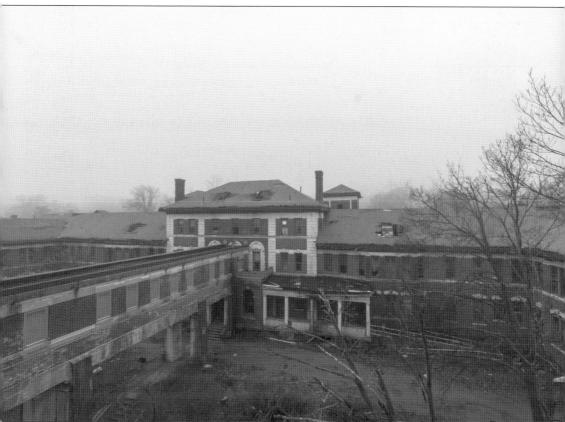

An iconic view of Hill Building 3, Rehabilitation Wards, was taken from the rooftop of Building 11, Reception Wards. This photograph shows the symmetry with which this building was constructed. Extending out from the center is the raised breezeway that connected the two buildings above ground. The porches that are seen on Hill Building 3 are referenced in the 1917 annual report book. The warden's report for that year suggests the building have porches added on for fresh-air treatment of recovering patients. The top floor of the center portion of Hill Building 3 housed the dental ward for the hospital. The tower-like structures extending from the roof behind the chimneys were added for ventilation purposes. The breezeway is the only piece of architecture in this photograph that is not original to the 1900s. (Photograph by Kevin Kowalick.)

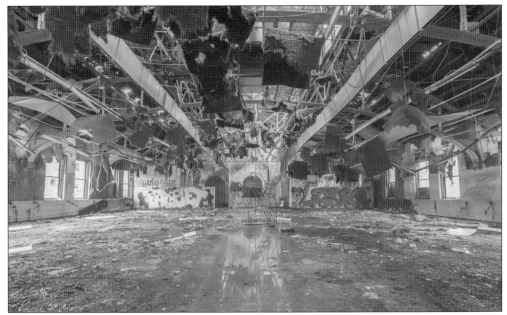

This photograph shows the female dining hall, Dining Hall 9. The modernized drop ceiling can be seen falling away and revealing the original architecture of this building. The kitchen hallway to transport food connected to the dining hall through the door seen behind the archway in the back center of the photograph. The building was in perfect condition after closure and fell quickly into disrepair due to neglect. (Photograph by Kevin Kowalick.)

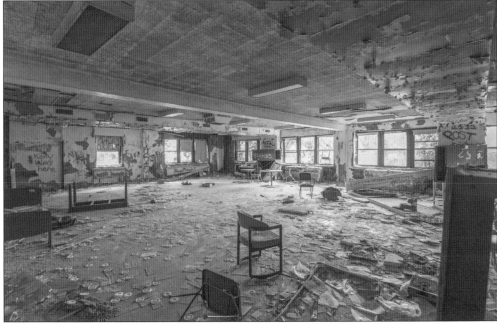

The top floor of Building 7, the Service Building, was used as conference room. After the demolition of the auditorium, county freeholders held meetings here regarding the hospital center. Directly below this room was the chapel. This room can be seen in use during an official meeting in chapter 4. (Photograph by Kevin Kowalick.)

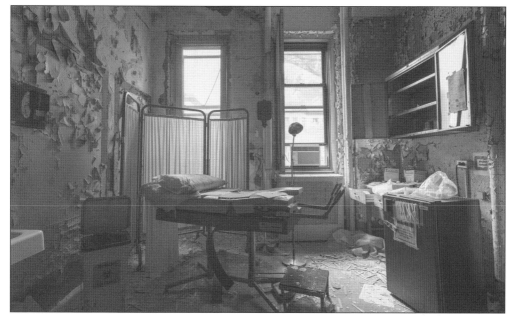

A gynecology office was inside Building 11, the Reception Wards. The examination offices were on the second floor. Being the largest building on the campus after demolition of the Star Building, it housed many different areas. Dayrooms, TV rooms, medical examination rooms, game rooms, laundry rooms, mass patient rooms, and staff offices were all located in the aboveground portion of this building. (Photograph by Kevin Kowalick.)

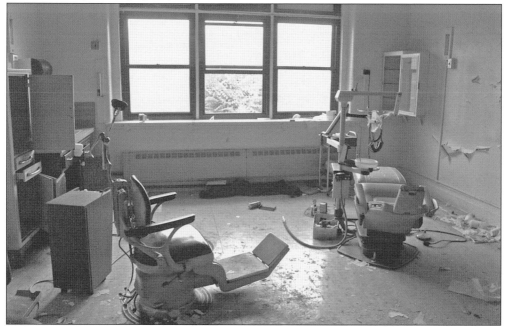

Overbrook's dentistry ward is seen in 2007 in Hill Building 3. In 1957, Overbrook was one of the first institutions in the country to obtain a new dentistry drill. This drill was the first non-hand-piece drill available since turn of the century. In 1957, the dentistry department had 3,573 visits with 1,065 extractions. (Photograph by Daniel Runyan.)

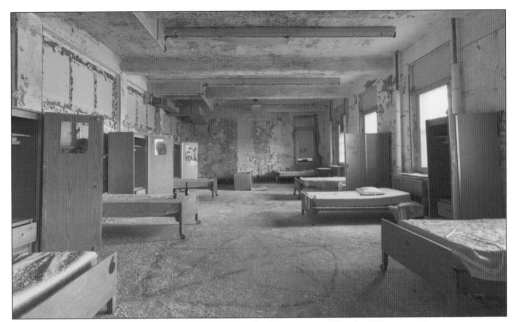

This example of a mass patient room was in the Reception Wards. These patient rooms were added to the existing 1925 structure in 1960. These rooms slept around seven to nine patients on average. During a period of severe overcrowding, the addition was made to free up some space in the existing building. (Photograph by Kevin Kowalick.)

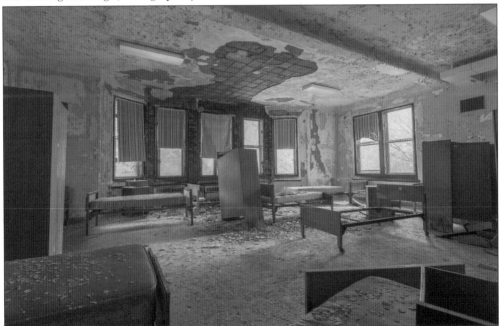

Another attempt at resolving overcrowding at Overbrook was converting dayrooms into patient housing. This solarium dayroom on the second floor of Hill Building 4, Front Male Wards, was outfitted with beds and wardrobes to accommodate patients. Most of the dayrooms on the first floor remained, but the second-floor dayrooms were converted into patient housing. (Photograph by Kevin Kowalick.)

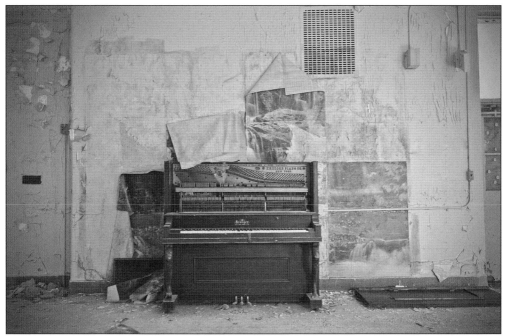

The first-floor dayrooms of the Hill Buildings still had some pianos remaining in them after closure. In this 2013 photograph, a piano from a dayroom inside Hill Building 2 remains in a state of decay. Many pianos inside the Hill Buildings were moved there from the Star Building after its demolition in the 1970s. (Photograph by Kathryn Cataldo.)

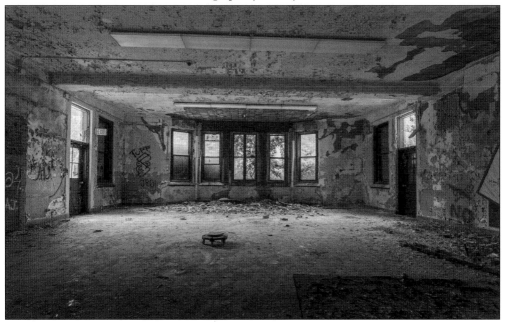

A typical solarium-style dayroom inside Hill Building 1 is seen after abandonment. This photograph can be compared to the photographs of these rooms in chapters 2 and 4. The architecture remains original from the 1900s, but most of the furniture was cleaned out of the rooms after closing. (Photograph by Kevin Kowalick.)

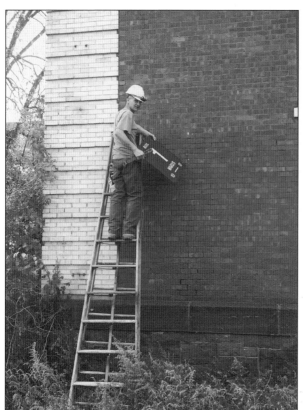

In 2016, Robert L. Williams and Mark Miller were given access to the hospital center in an effort to remove anything historical that could be preserved. This was the only effort put into preserving items from the hospital center. Author Kevin Kowalick was able to assist them in removing items from the hospital. In this photograph, Mark Miller removes a sign from Hill Building 1 to be saved. (Photograph by Kevin Kowalick.)

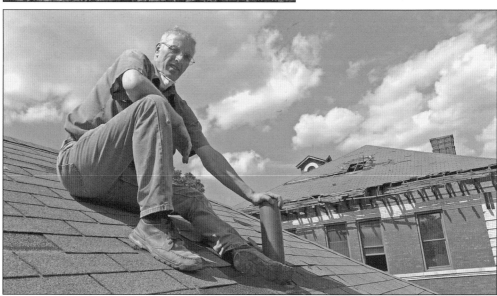

Robert L. Williams of the Verona Historical Society and longtime Verona resident has an extensive history with Overbrook. He has studied and visited Overbrook for many years. Robert has been able to single-handedly save some of the hospital's most historic items for preservation. His knowledge of the hospital center is outstanding, and the history of Overbrook can live on due to his efforts. (Photograph by Mark Miller.)

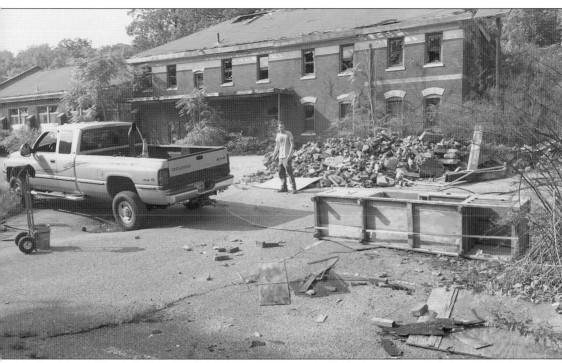

Author Kevin Kowalick helps Mark Miller remove an early-1900s dresser from Overbrook. Mark later restored this piece to outstanding condition. He has a special talent for being able to restore architectural pieces of Overbrook. Mark has saved everything from filing cabinets to the beautiful wooden columns of the Hill Building porches. When assisting Mark and Robert, author Kevin Kowalick discovered a cabinet of patient records in the basement of Hill Building 3. These records dated back to the 1890s, when the hospital was named Essex County Hospital for the Insane. Kevin, Robert, and Mark were able to pull all the records out of the basement for preservation. Robert cleaned and preserved the records, which were donated to the Cedar Grove Historical Society and the Verona Historical Society. (Photograph by Mark Miller.)

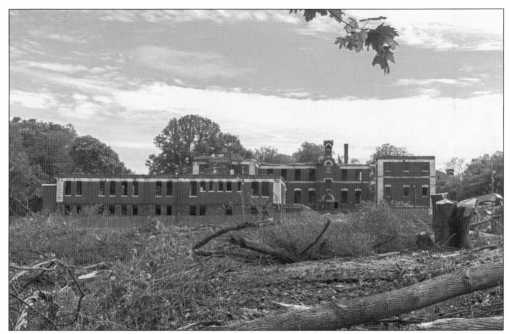

In 2016 and 2017, demolition rapidly progressed throughout the hospital center. The property was finally sold to K. Hovnanian after years of legal battles between Hovnanian and Essex County. The first Hill Building to be demolished was Five, the Back Male Wards. The Robert J. O'Toole Community Center now stands in the vicinity of where Hill Building 5 once stood. (Photograph by Kevin Kowalick.)

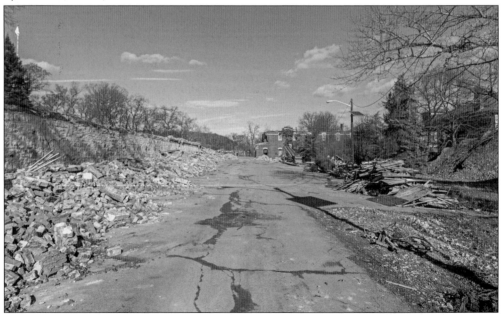

In the winter of 2017, the iconic kitchen hallway was demolished. This view shows the length of the kitchen hallway in rubble. The hallway looked exactly the same in the 1914 photograph in chapter 2 as it did the day before it was demolished. Shortly after this, the female dining hall was also demolished. (Photograph by Kevin Kowalick.)

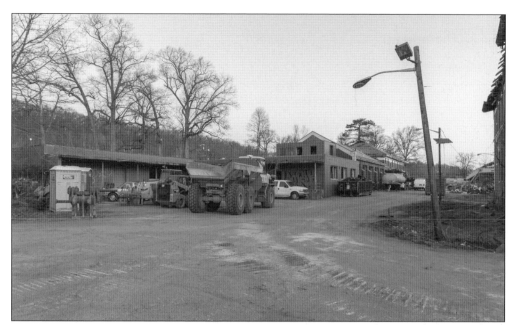

After the demolition of the kitchen hallway and dining room came the demolition of the kitchen. This photograph shows demolition and asbestos abatement crews getting ready to work on a cold morning in November 2016. Asbestos crews must come in and remove all asbestos and hazardous materials from the building before demolition crews can knock it down. (Photograph by Kevin Kowalick.)

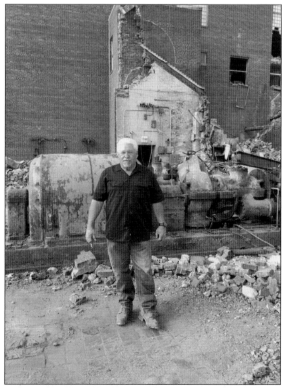

Dallas Construction Group was hired by K. Hovnanian to do the demolition work at Overbrook. Construction foreman Carl Franzetti is close with Robert, Mark, and Kevin and personally cares about the history of the hospital as much as they do. He and his team carefully remove key architectural elements from the buildings to be saved. Carl has played a large role in making sure the hospital is remembered after his job there is done. (Photograph by Robert L. Williams)

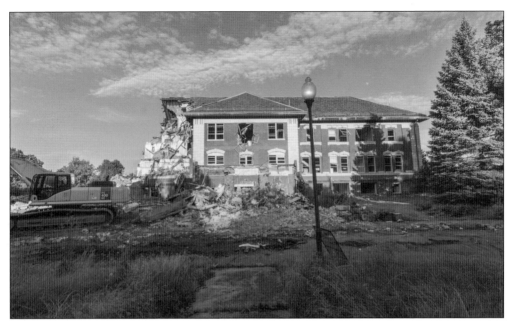

The Administration Building along Fairview Avenue was demolished in the summer of 2016. This building was easily recognizable by all who drove down the road. Here, the building can be seen in mid-demolition. The 1960s additions taken away, this view resembles the original building with the exception of the left half being partially destroyed. (Photograph by Kevin Kowalick.)

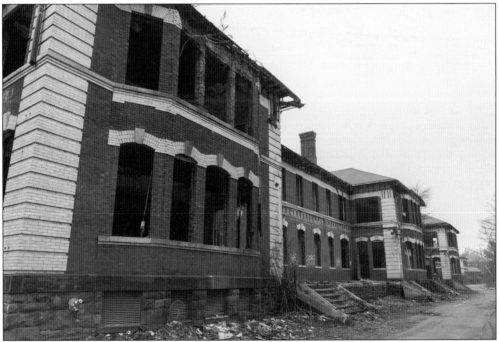

Hill Building 1, the Female Wards, was the second Hill Ward Building demolished. This photograph shows the building just before its destruction. The buildings were cleared of all their furniture and stripped of their architectural beauty. At that point, any asbestos needed to be removed and cleaned. After this, the building sits ready for demolition. (Photograph by Kevin Kowalick.)

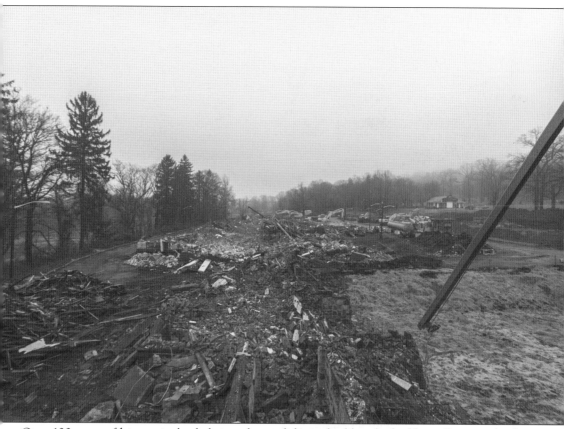

Over 100 years of history is slowly being chopped down, building by building. Great medical strides were made at Overbrook through the years that changed the way mental illness is treated today. A city within itself is slowly disappearing in Cedar Grove. The land is proposed to be rental condominiums, something that can be found around every corner in Northern New Jersey. Residents of Fairview Avenue are upset to see a large part of history destroyed and to have their neighborhood became even more overcrowded with the addition of these townhomes. The expansive woods around the complex are home to many types of wildlife. The large cedar trees will all be removed, with nothing saved to remember the hospital by. This photograph shows the footprint of Hill Building 1 after its complete removal. (Photograph by Kevin Kowalick.)

DISCOVER THOUSANDS OF LOCAL HISTORY BOOKS FEATURING MILLIONS OF VINTAGE IMAGES

Arcadia Publishing, the leading local history publisher in the United States, is committed to making history accessible and meaningful through publishing books that celebrate and preserve the heritage of America's people and places.

Find more books like this at
www.arcadiapublishing.com

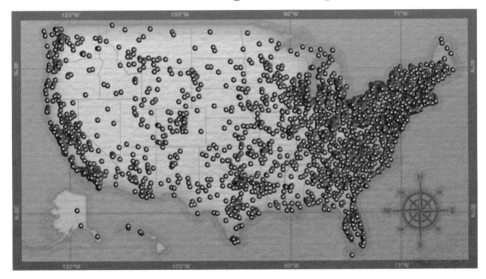

Search for your hometown history, your old stomping grounds, and even your favorite sports team.

Consistent with our mission to preserve history on a local level, this book was printed in South Carolina on American-made paper and manufactured entirely in the United States. Products carrying the accredited Forest Stewardship Council (FSC) label are printed on 100 percent FSC-certified paper.

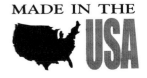

MADE IN THE
USA